REVISION IN SCIENCES BASIC TO OPHTHALMOLOGY

Raman Malhotra MB ChB

Senior House Officer,
The Western Eye Hospital, London

David Easty MB ChB MD FRCOphth

Professor & Head,
Department of Ophthalmology, Bristol University,
and Honorary Consultant
Bristol Eye Hospital, Bristol

A member of the Hodder Headline Group
LONDON • SYDNEY • AUCKLAND
Co-published in the USA by Oxford University Press, Inc., New York

First published in Great Britain in 1998 by
Arnold, a member of the Hodder Headline Group,
338 Euston Road, London NW1 3BH
http://www.arnoldpublishers.com

Co-published in the United States of America by
Oxford University Press, Inc.,
198 Madison Avenue, New York, NY 10016
Oxford is a registered trademark of Oxford University Press

Whilst the advice and information in this book is believed to be true and
accurate at the date of going to press, neither the author nor the publisher
can accept any legal responsibility or liability for any errors or omissions
that may be made.

British Library Cataloguing in Publication Data
A catalogue record for this book is available from the British Library

Library of Congress Cataloging-in-Publication Data
A catalog record for this book is available from the Library of Congress

ISBN 0 340 67678 7

Publisher: Georgina Bentliff
Production Editor: Liz Gooster
Production Controller: Sarah Kett

Typeset in 9/12pt Helvetica by J&L Composition Ltd, Filey, North Yorkshire
Printed and bound in Great Britain by J W Arrowsmith Ltd, Bristol

Dedicated to Kavita

CONTENTS

PREFACE

The examination in basic sciences towards the Fellowship of the Royal College of Ophthalmologists demands an in-depth knowledge of ophthalmic and general medical subjects including physiology, microbiology, pharmacology and anatomy. It is inevitable that in the course of preparation candidates will encounter new ocular concepts. There are few books available which were written specifically as revision texts, in other words presenting typical examination questions, model answers and clarification of difficult or important topics. This book, therefore, is aimed at meeting these objectives for candidates sitting the first part examination. It may also be useful to others who are preparing for related exams and wish to refresh their knowledge of certain topics.

The first part examination is divided into multiple choice question papers (MCQs) and essays. The MCQs cover an incredibly broad range of topics and test knowledge in quite fine detail. An MCQ is made up of 5 stems, each to be answered as being true or false. An incorrect answer carries the penalty of a mark deducted from those already scored. The essays however test the candidate's ability to offer a concise description or explanation of an issue with clarity of thought and structure. This method of examination challenges the candidate to acquire a depth of fine detailed knowledge yet at the same time maintain a clear overview of the subject.

This book consists of MCQs and diagrammatic essays. It occasionally but deliberately deviates from the examination MCQ format of 5 stems by including 6 or even 7 stems with the aim of offering practice to the reader. Along with the answers are included short explanatory notes on each subject that may be useful in preparing short note summaries.

The essays are of titles or subjects that are broad and open-ended, and their format allows their basic structure to be identified at a glance. Necessary background information is also included either in the summary page or further on. Essay answers require an appreciation of the question and an awareness of the priorities. To this end we have used a system of 'traffic lights' (red, amber and green) presented as black and white images in the essays. These serve as useful bullets both listing and prioritising key points. Red identifies the point or fact that is most important. Amber is attached to the second most important fact and green may signify either the third most important fact or (depending on its context) may indicate a point or feature of least importance. The 'traffic light' system allows facts to be grouped and then further listed (perhaps by number) in each group thereby avoiding the confusion of too many numbered points on a page. The system is for revision purposes only and has no place in essay answers. It is not universally used and may prove ambiguous to the examiner.

We hope that candidates sitting this exam will find this book useful, and for those who may be sitting their exam once again, do not despair, this is a well trodden path!

Raman Malhotra and David Easty
1997

ACKNOWLEDGEMENTS

We would like to thank the following individuals for their help in reviewing the manuscript:

Dr Neville Goodman
(Cardiovascular and Respiratory Physiology)
Senior Lecturer, Department of Anaesthesiology, University of Bristol

Dr Terry Hill
(Microbiology)
Reader in Microbiology, Department of Pathology and Microbiology, University of Bristol

Dr Graham Holder
(Electrophysiology)
Department of Electrodiagnostics, Moorfields Hospital, London

Dr Stephen Lisney
(Renal, Endocrine and Neurophysiology)
Head of Department, Department of Physiology, University of Bristol

Professor Gordon Ruskell
(Anatomy)
Department of Optometry and Visual Science, City University

Dr Edward Sheffield
(Pathology)
Senior Lecturer, Department of Pathology and Microbiology, University of Bristol

Mr Gary Shuttleworth
(Ocular Physiology and Pharmacology)
Lecturer, Department of Ophthalmology, University of Bristol

A special thank you to Gail Clare, Sue Tedd and Ann Young for typing the manuscript with such incredible patience.

INTRODUCTION

Universities and colleges set assessments to judge a level of achievement, to monitor progress, sometimes to motivate candidates and sometimes to license practice within a profession. Good assessments need to consider the mental and practical skills to be tested. In medicine the tests should be valid and determine levels of competence in a number of components. Factors that are important in assessment in medicine are recall of information, interpretation of data and problem-solving. Examinations should emulate relevant vocational conditions closely.

Assessment methods vary from the three-hour essay examination, through prepared essay exams, open book essays and short answer questions, to objective tests of various kinds including course work, practicals, simulated tasks and oral situations such as *viva voce* exams. In Part I of the MRCOphth Examination, basic science relevant to vision and the eye is evaluated. The methods involve a three-hour essay paper and two multiple choice papers. The former requires good knowledge of information, while the latter requires thought as well as information. The advantages of the multiple choice papers are that there is broad coverage of the syllabus, marking is objective and precise, and computer marking is possible.

What is the problem with these medical examinations, and why do candidates fail? What are the commonest errors in answering written questions? Does everybody pass the tests who should pass, or do unnecessary failures occur? Reasons for failure are many and varied. Given the motivation of those undertaking further training within the medical profession, it is unlikely that lack of ability or of hard work are factors. Thus the unsuccessful candidate may have other problems, such as social isolation, inadequate teaching and the pressure of medical training, together with lack of time for preparation. Overseas students may have difficulty with language and essay presentation; without good English, it is difficult to write an acceptable answer. There are many ways in which these problems can be alleviated. Simple suggestions to improve exam success include the following. Rehearse essay preparation questions before the exam since practice improves outcome. Do not just copy out facts from text books. Try to imitate examination conditions, and become expert in planning questions, and then writing them out in a measured time interval. Get a senior colleague to read through trial questions and invite him or her to review it critically. Everybody has their own method for preparation, but remember that over-preparation can lead to disaster. Do not use too many texts within the same field – stick with a readable one, and do not expand into reference texts. Make sure that you understand the science. In your preparation try to grasp the science of physiology, pathology, anatomy or biochemistry. Understanding helps in memorizing facts, and in explanations or descriptions in answers to questions.

What is the best technique to use to persuade examiners to give a pass mark? Adequate preparation is crucial. The pressure to continue quickly up the career ladder has always been considerable and there is often a tendency to enter a exam too early. Premature entry without adequate preparation rarely results in a successful outcome. Cover the total subject matter during this period. Presentation of essays is fundamental for success. Be careful to write legibly, and avoid clumsy corrections and crossings out. Use headings liberally, highlighting key words and important facts.

Principles

- Try to relax before the examination. There is little point in a last minute struggle to cover an extensive field.
- Read the instruction sheets and questions extremely carefully. All too frequently candidates misinterpret a question, or lose marks by not following instructions. For example, candidates asked to answer three out of four short note questions, may answer only one. This is unfortunate, but will lose marks.
- Work out the time you must allocate to each question. Prepare a plan in about 10 minutes at the beginning. Make a skeleton answer with a series of headings. Avoid repetition. Try to convey a logical train of thought.
- Do not feel that you have to commit everything you know to paper – this will probably take far too long, and you will not have time to answer the other questions properly.
- Write legibly. Do not rush so that your script is indecipherable. A short answer that is readable is better than a long answer in an illegible scrawl.
- Try to be grammatically correct. Do not write in note form unless this is requested. Write in sentences. It is useful to itemize points, or related paragraphs as it demonstrates a well-organized approach. It may be useful to the examiners to underline in colour important points that you wish to highlight.
- Illustrations are regarded as helpful, but be careful – errors can be costly. If you are not certain of the facts, use description. If you decide to use a diagram, then take care and keep it neat and tidy. Casual thumb-nail sketches do not help very much.
- Flow diagrams, on the other hand, may shorten the text and provide the examiners with an idea of your train of thought.
- Avoid tables.
- Avoid abbreviations without explanation. Use them only after they have been explained, e.g. visual evoked response (VER). Very common abbreviations are permissible, such as IOP (intra-ocular pressure). If there is any doubt, write it out in full.
- Make the essay interesting. Do not make things up. Do not waffle. Short sentences are better than long ones.
- Give yourself time to read through the entire script at the end, so that errors can be corrected.
- Finally, try to be neat and tidy. Crossing out and sloppy presentation does not score points. The neatest writers score the most points in the end.

Our aim in this book is to provide help on the best way to answer an essay question. It also provides a series of multiple choice questions (MCQs) so that potential candidates can gain experience in this method of testing.

- Remember that if the answer to an MCQ is not known, do not try to guess the answer.

- Do not feel that you must answer all the questions; the examiners may use negative marking, i.e. an incorrect answer will lose a mark.
- Blanks do not lose marks. Pick out the questions that you really know first, and then see how much you have answered.

Examinations are regarded by some as a competition, to which candidates react in a number of ways. Thus studying past papers, doing practice answers as essays or multiple choice questions and so on are distinct from the disinterested pursuit of the subject to be studied. For example, essay questions may sometimes concern subjects that have been discussed at a national meeting. Topical issues are good subjects for questions. However some may feel that this is not a reasonable way to proceed, and therefore ignore this on principle. Others will depend on hard work alone. The greatest success comes from cue-consciousness and hard work. We hope that the examples of essay questions and MCQs in this book will help candidates towards a successful outcome.

Anatomy
Questions

1 In the orbital cavity,

   A the lateral wall of the cavity is directly related to the temporal fossa
   B the lateral wall of the orbit is made up of the zygomatic bone and the greater wing of the sphenoid only
   C the roof of the orbit is made up of the orbital plate of the frontal bone and the greater and lesser wings of the sphenoid
   D the frontal nerve is directly related to the entire length of the roof of the orbit
   E the medial wall of the orbit is made up by the frontal process of the maxilla, the lacrimal bone, the orbital plate of the ethmoid and the orbital process of the palatine bone

2 Which of the following statements regarding the orbital cavity are true?

   A Direct relations of the medial wall of the orbit include the sphenoid sinus, medial rectus and lacrimal sac.
   B The floor of the orbit is directly related to the inferior rectus.
   C The superior orbital fissure is closed laterally by the frontal bone.
   D The superior orbital fissure connects the orbital cavity with the pterygopalatine fossa.
   E The optic canal lies in the body of the sphenoid.
   F The optic canal is directed forwards, laterally and downwards.

3 The periorbita is firmly attached to the

   A orbital margins
   B orbital surface of the maxilla
   C sutures
   D lacrimal fossa
   E superior orbital fissure

4 Regarding the paranasal sinuses,

   A the maxillary sinus lies above the anterior five teeth
   B the maxillary sinus drains into the bulla ethmoidalis

C the frontal sinus drains into the hiatus semilunaris

D the lymphatic drainage of the posterior ethmoidal sinus is to the submandibular lymph nodes

E the frontal sinuses are the only sinuses not present at birth

F the sphenoidal sinus is related posteriorly to the pons

5 Which of the following statements about the eyelids are true?

A The nerves to the eyelids lie anterior to orbicularis.

B The lower tarsal plate is 5 mm in height at the middle and 1 mm thick.

C The medial palpebral ligament is attached to the posterior lacrimal crest.

D The lateral palpebral ligament is attached to the marginal tubercle 11 mm below the frontozygomatic suture.

E The lateral palpebral ligament lies anterior to the lateral palpebral raphé.

6 The orbital septum

A marks the junction between periosteum and periorbita

B lies behind the lateral palpebral ligament

C attaches behind the posterior lacrimal crest

D lies anterior to the medial palpebral ligament

E is pierced by an extension of the inferior rectus sheath

F is pierced by the lacrimal, supraorbital, supratrochlear and infraorbital nerves

7 Regarding the eyelids,

A the meibomian glands lie between the tarsal plate and the conjunctivae

B the glands of Moll are more numerous in the upper lid

C there are approximately two glands of Zeis to each cilium

D the arterial arches run anterior to orbicularis

E the marginal arterial arch runs 1 mm from the free margin of the eyelids

F the lymphatics of the upper eyelid drain to the preauricular nodes and the lower lid to the submandibular nodes

8 Which of the following statements about the eyelids are true?

A The orbital portion of orbicularis arises from the bony orbital margin medial to the supraorbital notch and the infraorbital foramen.

B The skin of the eyelid is separated from the palpebral portion of orbicularis by fat.

C The lacrimal portion of orbicularis arises from the posterior lacrimal crest.

D The subtarsal sulcus lies half way between the anterior and posterior edge of the lid margin.

E The grey line marks an avascular plane separating the tarsal plate from the conjunctiva.

9 Regarding the conjunctiva,

A the superior fornix of the conjunctiva lies 10 mm from the limbus

B the lateral conjunctival fornix lies 5 mm from the limbus

C the anterior conjunctival artery arises mainly from the palpebral arterial arches

D the conjunctiva fuses with Tenon's capsule 3 mm behind the limbus

E goblet cells are most concentrated in the upper temporal conjunctival fornix

F the superior peripheral arterial arch supplies blood to the largest area of conjunctiva

10 In the lacrimal system

A the lacrimal gland is situated superomedial to the globe

B basal tear flow is mainly drained by the nasolacrimal duct

C the orbital portion of the lacrimal gland is three times larger than the palpebral portion

D the orbital portion of the lacrimal gland is related inferiorly to the conjunctiva and globe

E the palpebral portion of the lacrimal gland is related anteriorly to the orbital septum

11 Which of the following statements about the lacrimal gland are true?

A The lacrimal gland is surrounded by a capsule.

B Excision of the palpebral portion of the lacrimal gland stops tear secretion almost completely.

C The lacrimal vein joins the ophthalmic vein.

D The lymphatic drainage of the lacrimal gland is to the preauricular nodes.

E Preganglionic parasympathetic innervation is via the lesser petrosal nerve.

12 In the lacrimal system,

A the lower lacrimal punctum is 6.5 mm from the medial canthus

B the superior lacrimal canaliculus is shorter than the inferior canaliculus

C the canaliculi pierce the lacrimal sac 5 mm below the apex of the lacrimal sac

D the normal diameter of the lacrimal canaliculus is 0.5 mm

E the lacrimal canaliculi are lined by stratified squamous epithelium

13 With regard to the lacrimal system,

    A the lacrimal sac is related medially to the anterior ethmoidal air cells and middle meatus of the nose

    B the angular vein crosses the medial palpebral ligament 8 mm from the medial canthus

    C the medial palpebral ligament lies over the lower two-thirds of the lacrimal sac

    D the nasolacrimal duct is 12 mm long

    E the nasolacrimal duct passes downwards, forwards and laterally

    F the nasolacrimal duct is lined by stratified squamous epithelium

14 Concerning the anatomy of the eyeball, which of the following are true?

    A The normal anteroposterior diameter of the adult globe is 24 mm.

    B The vertical diameter is greater than the horizontal diameter of the globe.

    C The globe lies inferolaterally in the orbital cavity.

    D One-third of the globe lies in front of the plane between the medial and lateral orbital margins.

    E The anteroposterior axis of the globe passes through the optic disc.

15 In the cornea,

    A the posterior radius of curvature is 7.5 mm

    B the peripheral cornea is more curved than the central cornea

    C the refractive power is mainly due to the curvature of the posterior surface

    D the refractive index is 1.33

    E the periphery is 1 mm thick

16 Which of the following statements about the cornea are correct?

    A The epithelium is 10% of the corneal thickness.

    B The superficial layer of cells is not more than one cell thick.

    C The basal layer consists of a single layer of tall columnar stem cells.

    D Bowman's membrane is 15–20 μm thick.

    E Bowman's membrane does not contain fibroblasts.

17 In the cornea,

    A Descemet's membrane is the endothelial basement membrane

    B the posterior layer of Descemet's membrane increases thickness throughout life

    C Bowman's membrane continues beyond the limbus as Schwalbe's line

D the endothelial layer of the cornea stops abruptly at the limbus

E the corneal endothelium is a bilayer of flat, hexagonal-shaped cells

18 The sclera

A is 0.6 mm thick at the equator

B is 0.3 mm thick just behind the insertion of the recti

C has four middle apertures found 4 mm in front of the equator

D has posterior apertures which transmit the long and short ciliary nerves and vessels

E contains an endothelial canal called the canal of Schlemm

19 Which of the following statements about the sclera are true?

A The scleral fibres anterior to the equator are directed longitudinally.

B The episclera is a highly vascular zone of loose connected tissue that becomes thinner towards the back of the eye.

C The lamina cribrosa is the weakest part of the sclera.

D The sclera has a rich sensory innervation.

E Type IV collagen is found mainly at the lamina cribrosa.

20 Regarding the sclera, which of the following are true?

A the sclera is one-third water and two-thirds protein.

B Bruch's membrane forms the inner layer of the sclera.

C the long posterior ciliary arteries enter the sclera 3.6 mm and 3.9 mm nasal and temporal to the optic nerve.

D the optic nerve pierces the sclera 3 mm medial to the mid-line and 1 mm above the horizontal meridian.

E The sclera increases in thickness with age.

21 The ciliary body

A is larger on the nasal side than the temporal side

B on the nasal side has a posterior border that lies 5 mm behind the corneoscleral limbus

C begins 1.5 mm behind the corneoscleral limbus in the vertical meridian

D contains the pars plicata which has an anteroposterior length of between 3.5 and 4 mm

E includes the pars plicata, which is made up of 20–30 folds, forming the ciliary process

22 In the ciliary body,

  A both pigmented and non-pigmented ciliary epithelia are cuboidal in the young
  B the blood aqueous barrier is formed by tight junctions at the basolateral surface of the non-pigmented epithelial cells
  C The pigmented epithelium forms the inner layer of the ciliary epithelium
  D at gap junctions, the non-pigmented epithelial cells are separated by 2 mm clefts
  E the greatest number of ciliary epithelial gap junctions occur between the pigmented and non-pigmented epithelia

23 Which of the following statements about the ciliary body are true?

  A Zonulae occludentes are not found between adjacent ciliary pigmented epithelial cells.
  B The pigmented epithelial cells contain fewer mitochondria than the non-pigmented epithelial cells.
  C The pigmented epithelial cells contain a greater degree of rough endoplasmic reticulum than the non-pigmented epithelial cells.
  D The non-pigmented epithelial basement membrane is continuous with the internal limiting membrane of the retina.
  E Capillaries in the ciliary stroma have discontinuous walls.

24 In the ciliary body,

  A the oblique ciliary muscle fibres make up the outermost fibres of the ciliary muscle
  B ciliary muscle contains more extensive mitochondria and endoplasmic reticulum than normal smooth muscle
  C the blood supply is derived from the continuation of the choriocapillaris
  D venous drainage body is mainly by the anterior ciliary vessels
  E parasympathetic, sympathetic and sensory innervation is received

25 Which of the following statements regarding the iris are true?

  A The iris and pupillary diameters measured through the cornea are magnified by 12%.
  B The iris is thickest at the ciliary margin.
  C The anterior surface of the iris is made up of a thin endothelial cell layer.
  D The stroma contains mast cells.
  E The stroma is rich in collagen and elastic fibres.
  F The fenestrated arterial vessels of the iris run in the stroma.

26 In the iris,

A the sphincter pupillae muscle is 1 mm wide
B the sphincter pupillae muscle is only found at the pupillary zone
C the dilator pupillae is made up of striated muscle fibres
D the dilator pupillae lies between the pupillary zone and the periphery of the iris
E the posterior pigment epithelium of the iris gives rise to the dilator pupillae muscle

27 With regard to the epithelium of the iris, which of the following are true?

A The posterior pigment epithelium is continuous with the non-pigmented epithelium of the ciliary body.
B The anterior epithelial cells are larger than the posterior epithelial cells.
C The posterior epithelial cells are more pigmented than the anterior epithelial cells.
D The posterior epithelial cells are columnar when the pupil is dilated.
E The pigmented epithelial cells oppose each other base-to-apex.

28 The lens

A has a radius of curvature at the posterior surface of 6 mm
B anterior surface lies 3 mm from the posterior surface of the cornea
C diameter is 10 mm
D is 3 mm thick in the adult
E has an epithelium made up of a bilayer of cells

29 Which of the following statements about the lens are true?

A The anterior lens capsule is thicker than the posterior capsule.
B The epithelial cells of the lens are columnar.
C The foetal nucleus is made up of 'Y-shaped' sutures.
D The anterior radius of curvature becomes smaller with age.
E Zonular fibres of the lens attach the capsule at the lens equator to the ciliary processes of the pars plicata as well as the pars plana.

30 In the choroid,

A the arterial blood supply is by the anterior as well as the long and short posterior ciliary arteries
B the short posterior ciliary arteries pierce the sclera within a 2.5 mm radius of the optic disc

C innervation is by the long and short ciliary nerves only

D parasympathetic innervation from the facial nerve is seen

E the suprachoroidal space is greatest seen at the macula

31 Regarding the choroid, which of the following are true?

A The choroid is thickest at the equator.

B Melanocytes are most densely found in the inner layers of the choroid.

C Veins form the majority of vessels in the choroid.

D Choroidal veins are most concentrated at the macula.

E The choriocapillaris lies sclerad to Bruch's membrane.

32 In the choroid,

A the endothelium of the arteries and arterioles is continuous

B the choriocapillaris is lined by a single layer of smooth muscle cells

C Bruch's membrane forms the inner layer of the choroid

D Bruch's membrane is continuous with the basement membrane of the retinal pigment epithelium

E Bruch's membrane is thickest anterior to the equator

33 Regarding the retina,

A the foveola is 3 mm from the temporal margin of the optic disc and 0.8 mm superior to its centre

B the fovea has the same diameter as the optic disc

C the retina is thinnest at the fovea

D the retina is thickest at the perifoveal region

E rods are absent within a radius of 2.8 mm from the centre of the foveola

34 In the retina,

A the fovea contains one-sixtieth of the entire retinal cones

B there are approximately 120 000 000 rods

C the cones at the foveola are not separated from each other by Müller cells

D regarding the cone photoreceptor, the outer membrane of the outer segment is discontinuous with the discs

E the connecting stalk of the photoreceptor contains 10 pairs of microtubules and no central pair

35 Which of the following statements about the retina are true?

   A The ellipsoid is the outer portion of the photoreceptor inner segment.
   B The ellipsoid is predominantly rich in rough endoplasmic reticulum.
   C The outer nuclear layer lies between the external limiting membrane and the outer plexiform layer.
   D The external limiting membrane is made of up of a continuous row of zonulae occludentes.
   E The outer plexiform layer lies between the outer nuclear layer and the external limiting membrane.

36 With regard to the retina,

   A ganglion cells do not exist at the fovea or optic disc
   B Müller cells extend from the external limiting lamina to the internal limiting lamina
   C the internal limiting lamina is formed by a continuous row of zonulae adherentes between Müller cell processes
   D the retinal arteries are only found in the nerve fibre layer
   E the central retinal vein lies medial to the central retinal artery at the optic disc
   F the retinal capillaries do not pass towards the sclera beyond the inner nuclear layer

37 Which of the following statements about the retina are true?

   A Retinal capillaries consist of non-fenestrated endothelium and pericytes outside the endothelium.
   B Retinal pigment epithelial cells at the macula are taller and contain more melanin than those in the retinal periphery.
   C The basement membrane of the retinal pigment epithelium is continuous with that of the ciliary pigment epithelium.
   D Retinal pigment epithelial cells are attached to each other at their basolateral surfaces by zonulae occludentes and zonulae adherentes.
   E Retinal arteries are two-thirds to three-quarters the diameter of retinal veins.

38 The extraocular muscles: regarding the rectus muscles,

   A the superior rectus is the longest rectus muscle
   B the inferior rectus is the shortest rectus muscle
   C the lateral rectus has the longest tendon length
   D the medial rectus inserts into the sclera closest to the limbus
   E the rectus muscles are each approximately 40 mm in length

39 Which of the following statements about the extraocular muscles are true?

A The tendon of the superior oblique hooks through the trochlea and inserts into the sclera 54° to the sagittal plane.

B The superior oblique passes above the superior rectus.

C The inferior oblique passes above the inferior rectus.

D The inferior rectus sheath also inserts into the lower lid.

E The medial rectus is innervated by the superior division of the oculomotor nerve.

40 With regard to the arteries and nerves serving the extraocular muscles,

A the lacrimal artery lies inferior to the lateral rectus

B the ophthalmic artery lies superior to the medial rectus

C the ophthalmic artery passes below the superior rectus

D the superior division of the oculomotor nerve pierces levator before terminating in the superior rectus

E the trochlea nerve pierces the superior oblique close to its insertion

41 The orbital blood vessels: the ophthalmic artery

A arises medial to the anterior clinoid process and below the optic nerve

B lies within the dural sheath throughout its course in the optic canal

C lies medial to the ciliary ganglion in the orbital cavity

D divides terminally into the medial palpable artery and the dorsal nasal artery

E arises from the internal carotid artery and lies in the subdural space before reaching the optic canal

F occasionally enters the orbital cavity through the superior orbital fissure

42 Which of the following statements about the orbital blood vessels are true?

A The central retinal artery enters the inferomedial surface of the optic nerve.

B The lacrimal artery follows the lacrimal nerve in the orbital cavity above the lateral rectus.

C The anterior ethmoidal artery supplies the dura of the anterior fossa, anterior and middle ethmoidal sinuses and the frontal sinus.

D The posterior ethmoidal artery is a branch of the nasociliary artery.

E Anterior ciliary arteries arise from the muscular arteries.

43 The tributaries of the cavernous sinus include

 A the superior ophthalmic vein
 B the central retinal vein
 C the sphenoparietal sinus
 D the pterygoid plexus
 E the superior petrosal sinus

44 Regarding the veins,

 A the cavernous sinus extends from the superior orbital fissure to the apex of the petrous temporal bone
 B the central retinal vein leaves the optic nerve 12.5 mm from the eyeball
 C the superior ophthalmic vein receives blood from the central retinal vein
 D the inferior ophthalmic vein lies above the inferior rectus and communicates with the pterygoid plexus
 E the cavernous sinus lies medial to the trigeminal ganglion

45 Which of the following statements about the visual pathway are correct?

 A The intraorbital optic nerve is up to 30 mm long.
 B The optic chiasma commonly lies 10 mm directly above the dorsum sellae.
 C Fibres of the inferior nasal retina are related to the posterior portion of the optic chiasma.
 D The arterial blood supply to the intracranial portion of the optic nerve is by the superior hypophyseal and ophthalmic arteries.
 E Ventromedial fibres of the optic tract correspond to the superior contralateral visual field.
 F Macular fibres of the retina correspond to the ventromedial fibres of the optic tract.

46 Regarding the visual pathway,

 A superior retinal fibres correspond to medial cells at the lateral geniculate nucleus
 B ipsilateral temporal retinal fibres synapse in layers 2, 4 and 5 of the lateral geniculate nucleus
 C macular fibres of the retina correspond to the most medial portion of the lateral geniculate nucleus
 D superior retinal fibres correspond to fibres in the superior lip of the calcarine sulcus
 E fibres of the optic radiation relating to the inferior retinal quadrants are related inferolaterally to the anterior tip of the temporal horn of the lateral ventricle

47 With regard to the ventricles,

  A the lateral wall of the third ventricle is formed by the thalamus
  B the aqueduct of Sylvius is a communication between the third ventricle and each lateral ventricle
  C the only ports of exit for cerebrospinal fluid in the ventricles are the foramina of Magendie and Luschka
  D the roof of the anterior horn of the lateral ventricle is formed by the corpus callosum
  E the thalamus forms the medial wall of the body of the lateral ventricle
  F the optic radiations lie in the lateral wall of the posterior horn of the lateral ventricle

48 Which of the following statements about the oculomotor nerve are true?

  A The oculomotor nerve emerges from the mid-brain lateral to the cerebral peduncles.
  B Section of the third nerve causes lacrimation.
  C The ciliary ganglion is enclosed in dura.
  D The oculomotor complex innervates the ipsilateral inferior rectus, medial rectus and superior rectus.
  E The nerve to the inferior oblique muscle is responsible for supplying myelinated preganglionic parasympathetic fibres to the ciliary ganglion.

49 The trochlear nerve

  A is the thinnest cranial nerve
  B lies dorsomedial to the medial longitudinal fasciculus
  C the IV nucleus is connected by the medial longitudinal fasciculus to the III, V and VIII nuclei
  D supplies the contralateral superior oblique muscle
  E enters the orbital cavity outside the common tendinous ring
  F passes medially below levator in the orbital cavity to pierce the superior oblique muscle

50 Which of the following statements about the trigeminal nerve are true?

  A Fibres from the ophthalmic root lie ventrolaterally in the spinal tract of the trigeminal nerve.
  B The frontal nerve is the largest branch of the ophthalmic division.
  C The trigeminal nerve is responsible for the oculocardiac reflex.

D The maxillary division supplies sensory innervation to the face via the infraorbital zygomaticofacial and zygomaticotemporal nerves only.

E The buccal nerve carries sensory innervation to the cheek and is a branch of the maxillary division.

F The auriculotemporal nerve supplies sensory innervation to the parotid fascia.

51 The abducent nerve

A carries parasympathetic fibres

B innervates the ipsilateral lateral rectus

C runs lateral to and parallel with the internal carotid artery in the cavernous sinus

D receives sympathetic fibres in the cavernous sinus from the internal carotid plexus, which then leave to join the ophthalmic division of the trigeminal nerve

E leaves the brainstem at the lower border of the mid-brain

52 Which of the following statements about the facial nerve are true?

A The chorda tympani carries somatic afferent innervation to the anterior two-thirds to the tongue.

B The facial nerve supplies motor innervation to stapedius distal to the geniculate ganglion.

C The posterior auricular nerve is a branch of the facial nerve.

D The chorda tympani supplies preganglionic parasympathetic fibres to the sub-mandibular ganglion.

E The greater petrosal nerve leaves the main facial nerve at the geniculate ganglion.

F The greater petrosal nerve carries taste fibres from both the hard and soft palates.

53 In the face and scalp,

A the pterygomandibular raphé consists of interdigitating fibres of buccinator and middle constrictor

B buccinator is a muscle of mastication innervated by the mandibular division of the trigeminal nerve

C the internal and external carotid arteries anastomose at the junction of the forehead and the temple

D terminal branches of the superficial temporal artery enter the orbit through the inferior orbital fissure

E blood vessels of the scalp run in the loose areolar tissue between the aponeurosis and the pericranium

F temporalis and medial pterygoid retract the mandible

54 Which of the following statements about the thyroid gland are correct?

A The thyroid gland lies behind the pretracheal fascia.
B The isthmus lies in front of the second, third and fourth tracheal rings.
C The inferior thyroid artery arises from the branch of the first part of subclavian artery.
D The arterial blood supplies to the upper and lower parathyroid glands are by the inferior thyroid artery.
E The venous drainage of the thyroid gland is to the internal jugular vein.

55 The cervical sympathetic trunk

A lies anterior to the neck of the first rib
B runs medial to the vertebral artery in the root of the neck
C lies behind prevertebral fascia
D lies medial to the carotid sheath
E lies lateral to the vagus nerve
F section results in exophthalmos
G ends at the superior cervical ganglion, which lies anterior to the lateral mass of the atlas and axis
H carries preganglionic sympathetic fibres to synapse at the middle cervical ganglion, which lies anterior to the vertebral artery at the level of C6 vertebra.

56 Which of the following statements about cervical sympathetic innervation are true?

A Postganglionic fibres from the superior cervical ganglion are distributed to C1–4.
B Postganglionic fibres from the inferior cervical ganglion are distributed to the vertebral artery.
C Only the middle cervical ganglion supplies fibres to the cardiac plexus.
D The inferior and middle cervical ganglia supply fibres to the hand.
E The trachea receives sympathetic innervation from the middle cervical ganglion.

57 In the parotid region,

A the parotid gland is supplied by the VII nerve
B the marginal mandibular artery emerges at the lower border of the mandible anterior to the insertion of masseter
C the capsule of the parotid gland is derived from the investing layer of deep cervical fascia
D the parotid duct arises from the gland deep to the branches of the facial nerve
E preauricular lymph nodes exist deep to the parotid capsule and within the parotid gland

F the parotid duct pierces masseter and buccinator to open into the cheek

G the parotid duct opens opposite the second upper premolar tooth

58 With regard to the cerebral vessels, which of the following statements are true?

A The posterior cerebral artery is a branch of the internal carotid artery.

B The anterior communicating artery supplies the optic chiasma.

C The anterior cerebral artery supplies arterial blood to motor and sensory areas of the contralateral leg, the perineum, micturition and defaecation centres.

D The circle of Willis is formed by the internal carotid and basilar arteries only.

E Occlusion of the middle cerebral artery may result in a contralateral weakness of the lower portion of the face.

59 Regarding the cerebral vessels,

A the anterior cerebral artery passes above the optic nerve and runs in the longitudinal fissure

B the posterior cerebral artery runs beneath the tentorium cerebelli

C the middle cerebral artery supplies 90% of the visual cortex

D the posterior communicating artery is the main supply to the anterior third of the optic radiation

E occlusion of the basilar artery results in bilateral paralysis

60 In the cerebral vessels,

A the posterior cerebral artery supplies the posterior portion of the optic radiation

B occlusion of the posterior cerebral artery produces a contralateral homonymous hemianopia

C the anterior choroidal and posterior communicating arteries are the main source of arterial supply to the optic tract

D The middle cerebral artery is the largest branch of the internal carotid artery

E The middle cerebral artery runs in the lateral sulcus

ANATOMY
Answers

1 **A** = True   **B** = True   **C** = False   **D** = True   **E** = False

The lateral wall of the orbit is made up of the zygomatic bone, including the marginal tubercle of Whitnall (Professor of Anatomy at McGill University in Montreal and Bristol University) and the greater wing of the sphenoid. Anteriorly it is directly related to the temporal fossa and further back, to the middle cranial fossa.

The roof of the orbit is a triangular plate consisting of the orbital part of the frontal bone and the lesser wing of the sphenoid. Throughout its length, the roof is directly related to the frontal nerve. The medial wall is the thinnest wall of the orbit (less than 0.4 mm). It consists of the frontal process of the maxilla, the lacrimal bone, the orbital plate of the ethmoid and the body of the sphenoid.

2 **A** = True   **B** = True   **C** = True   **D** = False   **E** = False   **F** = True

The direct medial relation of the medial wall of the orbit includes the nasal cavity, ethmoid sinuses and sphenoid sinus. It is posteriorly related to the optic canal. The medial wall is also directly related to the medial rectus, superior oblique, anterior and posterior ethmoidal nerves, infratrochlear nerve and the termination of the ophthalmic artery. It is related anteriorly to the lacrimal sac (lying in the lacrimal fossa). The apex of the floor of the orbit is directly related above to the inferior rectus muscles. Further forward the two are separated by inferior oblique as well as orbital fat.

The superior orbital fissure is formed by the greater and lesser wings of the sphenoid and is closed laterally by the frontal bone. It lies between the roof and the lateral wall of the orbit and connects the orbital cavity with the middle cranial fossa.

The inferior orbital fissure is bounded by the greater wing of the sphenoid posteriorly, and by the maxilla and orbital processes of the palatine bone and anteriorly. It connects the orbital cavity with the pterygopalatine fossa and thus the infratemporal fossa.

The optic canal lies in the lesser wing of the sphenoid and is directed forward, laterally and downwards.

3 **A** = True   **B** = False   **C** = True   **D** = True   **E** = True

The periorbita, or orbital periosteum, lines the orbital cavity. It is firmly attached to the orbital margins, sutures, fissures and foramina and the lacrimal fossa. It is loosely attached to the bony surface.

4 **A** = False **B** = False **C** = True **D** = False **E** = True **F** = True

The maxillary sinus of Highmore (seventeenth-century physician of Sherborne) lies above the posterior five teeth (two premolars, three molars). The roots of these teeth often protrude into the sinus. The ostium of the sinus opens into the middle meatus in the hiatus semilunaris. The frontal sinus drains by the infundibulum into the hiatus semilunaris of the middle meatus. The sphenoidal sinus and posterior ethmoidal sinus lymphatic drainage is to the retropharyngeal lymph nodes. The remaining sinuses drain to the submandibular nodes.

The paranasal sinuses arise as outbuddings of the nasal mucosa. The frontal sinus is the only sinus not present at birth. It may be thought of as an anterior ethmoidal air cell that has migrated forwards. It appears in the second year and does not reach full size until approximately 25 years of age. The sphenoidal sinus is related anteriorly to the ethmoidal sinus and the nose, laterally to the cavernous sinus, internal carotid artery and abducent nerve, posteriorly to the posterior cranial fossa and the pons, superiorly to the pituitary gland, optic nerve and chiasma and inferiorly to the pterygoid canal and nasopharynx.

5 **A** = False **B** = True **C** = False **D** = True **E** = True

The main nerves to the eyelid lie with the blood vessels posterior to orbicularis in front of the tarsal plate and orbital septum. The upper tarsal plate is between 10 and 11 mm in height in the middle. Its lateral edge is 7 mm from the marginal tubercle of Whitnall and the medial end is approximately 9 mm from the anterior lacrimal crest. The lower tarsal plate is 5 mm in height at the middle. Both tarsal plates are approximately 13 mm wide and 1 mm thick.

The medial palpebral ligament is a triangular ligament attached to the frontal process of the maxilla at the anterior lacrimal crest. It lies anterior to the lacrimal sac.

The lateral palpebral ligament lies behind the palpebral raphé of orbicularis and anterior to a lobule of the lacrimal gland and lateral check ligament.

6 **A** = True **B** = False **C** = True **D** = False **E** = True **F** = True

The orbital septum is attached along the orbital margin and marks the junction between periosteum and periorbita. It is continuous with the tarsal plate except where it is pierced by fibres of levator or an extension of the inferior rectus sheath inserting into the skin of the eyelid and border of the tarsal plate. The lateral side is superficial and medial side deep. It lies anterior to the lateral palpebral ligament, bridges the supraorbital notch forming the foramen, passes anterior to the trochlea, leaves the bone briefly and reattaches behind the posterior lacrimal crest, lacrimal sac and medial palpebral ligament but anterior to the medial check ligament.

The orbital septum is pierced by the lacrimal, supraorbital and supratrochlear vessels and nerves, the infratrochlear nerve, the anastomosis of the angular vein and the ophthalmic vein, medial palpebral arteries, fibres of levator and inferior rectus sheath.

7 **A** = False **B** = False **C** = True **D** = False **E** = False **F** = False

The meibomian glands lie actually in the tarsal plate but may be seen as yellow streaks through the conjunctivae of an everted eyelid. The glands of Moll (ciliary glands) are modified sweat glands that open either into a follicle, between two lashes or into a gland of Zeis duct. They are more numerous in the lower lid than upper. The glands of Zeis are modified sebaceous glands attached to ciliary follicles. Each cilium has two glands. Their oily secretions prevent desiccation of lashes and contribute to the tear film.

The blood supply to the eyelids is via the medial and lateral palpebral arteries (ophthalmic and lacrimal arteries). These form marginal and peripheral arches that run behind orbicularis and in front of the tarsal plate and pierce both orbicularis to supply structures anteriorly, and the tarsal plates to supply the palpebral conjunctiva.

The marginal arterial arch runs 3 mm from the free margin of the eyelids.

The lymphatics of the medial third of the upper and lower eyelids (including conjunctiva) follow the facial vein and drain to the submandibular nodes, whereas the lateral two-thirds drain to the preauricular and parotid nodes.

8 **A** = True **B** = False **C** = True **D** = False **E** = False

Orbicularis has three portions: an orbital, a palpebral, and a lacrimal portion. The palpebral portion may be divided into a pretarsal muscle (in front of the tarsal plate) and a preseptal muscle (in front of the orbital septum). The pretarsal muscle arises from the lateral palpebral ligament and sweeps medially to insert into the medial palpebral ligament. The preseptal muscle arises from the lateral palpebral ligament and also inserts into the medial palpebral ligament. Deep fibres insert into the lacrimal fascia of the lateral wall of the lacrimal sac. These fibres are thought to be responsible for the lacrimal sac 'vacuum effect'. The orbital portion arises from the medial orbital margin between the supraorbital notch (superiorly) down to the margin medial to the infraorbital foramen as well as the medial palpebral ligament.

Areolar tissue intervenes between the palpebral portion of orbicularis and the skin, as well as the tarsal plate. No fat exists here. The situation reverses with regards to the orbital portion of orbicularis where fat (and no areolar tissue) lies between the skin and the muscle. The lacrimal portion (Horner's muscle) is in the form of a thin layer of muscle arising from behind the lacrimal sac from the posterior lacrimal crest passing forward and lateral to the lacrimal sac before dividing into an upper and lower portion terminating at the medial margins of the upper and lower lids. It is often thought of as a deep portion of the pretarsal muscle, part of the palpebral portion of the orbicularis.

Approximately 2 mm from the posterior edge of the lid margin lies the subtarsal sulcus, a shallow groove providing an entry for perforating vessels from the eyelid as well as a trap for foreign particles.

On eversion of the eyelid, it is important to examine the sulcus in the search for foreign bodies. Approximately half way between the anterior and posterior edges of the lid margin is found the grey line that marks an avascular plane separating the tarsal plate from orbicularis. The lid may be split in this plane.

9 **A** = True **B** = False **C** = False **D** = True **E** = False **F** = True

The conjunctiva consists of a palpebral part, an orbital part and a fornix. The palpebral conjunctiva is firmly adherent to the entire width of the superior tarsal plate and half the lower tarsal plate. The conjunctival fornix has a superior, inferior, lateral and medial portion. The superior fornix is found 10 mm from the limbus. The inferior fornix lies 8 mm from the limbus. The lateral fornix lies 14 mm from the limbus (extending just behind the equator of the globe). The medial fornix is essentially absent due to the presence of the caruncle and plica semilunaris.

The bulbar conjunctiva is separated from Tenon's capsule up to 3 mm from the limbus by loose areolar tissue. Subconjunctival vessels may be found in this space. The conjunctiva fuses with Tenon's capsule 3 mm from the limbus .

The blood supply to the conjunctiva is from the palpebral arteries and the anterior ciliary arteries (continuations of the muscular arteries). The palpebral arteries form the marginal and peripheral arterial arches. The peripheral arterial arch of the upper lid supplies the largest area of conjunctiva, including the palpebral conjunctiva, the superior fornix and the bulbar conjunctiva up to approximately 4 mm from the limbus. The inferior peripheral arterial arch is often absent. The arterial arches give rise to the posterior conjunctival artery. The anterior ciliary artery gives rise to the anterior conjunctival artery. These two anastomose at around 4 mm from the limbus. Goblet cells are found all over the conjunctiva and deep in the epithelium. They are most concentrated inferonasally at the bulbar conjunctiva and least concentrated supratemporally in the fornix. They are absent at the nasal and temporal bulbar conjunctiva near the limbus.

10 **A** = False **B** = False **C** = True **D** = False **E** = False

The lacrimal system comprises the lacrimal gland superolateral to the globe producing tears, the lacrimal canaliculi, the lacrimal sac and nasolacrimal duct.

Under basal conditions of tear production tears are removed mainly by evaporation and virtually none passes down the nasolacrimal duct which exists along with the nasolacrimal sac to remove excess tears. The lacrimal gland is made up of a large orbital portion and a smaller palpebral portion. The orbital portion rests in the lacrimal fossa and is related superiorly to the fossa (frontal bone), inferiorly to levator, its tendon expansion and the lateral rectus, anteriorly to the orbital septum and posteriorly to the orbital fat.

The small palpebral portion lies superolateral to the superior conjunctival fornix. It is separated from the orbital portion above by levator.

11 **A** = True   **B** = True   **C** = True   **D** = True   **E** = False

The lacrimal gland is surrounded by a capsule. Its masses of lobules are often separated by the surrounding orbital fat.

Approximately five ducts pass from the orbital portion through the palpebral portion and about six in number drain to the superior conjunctival fornix. Due to this arrangement it is seen that excision of the palpebral portion of the lacrimal gland will reduce tear secretion to almost zero.

Arterial supply is mainly by the lacrimal artery but occasionally also by the infraorbital artery. Venous drainage is by the corresponding vein which drains into the ophthalmic vein. Lymphatic drainage is via the conjunctival lymphatics to the preauricular and parotid nodes.

The lacrimal gland receives both parasympathetic and sympathetic as well as sensory innervation. Parasympathetic innervation arises as preganglionic fibres from the superior salivatory nucleus via the nervus intermediate and from the geniculate ganglion to continue as the greater petrosal nerve passing through the petrous temporal bone and then entering a groove on its surface beneath the dura of the middle cranial fossa and the trigeminal ganglion. Running across the foramen lacerum it is joined by the postganglionic sympathetic fibres of the internal carotid plexus known as the deep petrosal nerve, and becomes the nerve of the pterygoid canal (Vidian's nerve). This nerve passes through the pterygoid canal to reach the pterygopalatine fossa and the preganglionic fibres synapse at the pterygopalatine ganglion. Postganglionic fibres are thought to either 'hitch-hike' via the zygomatic nerve zygomaticotemporal and lacrimal nerve, or, as described by Ruskell, probably reach directly by a retro-orbital plexus through the inferior orbital fissure to the lacrimal gland.

Sensory innervation is by the lacrimal nerve, a branch of the ophthalmic division of the trigeminal nerve. The lesser petrosal nerve carries preganglionic parasympathetic secretomotor fibres from the inferior salivary nucleus and the timpanic branch of the glossopharyngeal nerve. It is formed at the medial wall of the middle ear and leaves by passing up through the petrous temporal bone into the middle cranial fossa. It runs forward beneath the dura and leaves through the foramen ovale to synapse to the otic ganglion in the infratemporal fossa. Postganglionic parasympathetic fibres innervate the parotid gland.

12 **A** = True   **B** = True   **C** = False   **D** = True   **E** = True

Each lacrimal punctum lies on a raised papilla; the lower punctum lies 6.5 mm from the medial canthus and the superior punctum slightly medial at 6 mm from the medial canthus. The lacrimal canaliculi begin at the puncta and consist of a 2 mm vertical and 8 mm (upper canaliculus being slightly shorter) horizontal component. They pierce the lacrimal sac separately approximately 2.5 mm below the apex of the lacrimal sac. The normal diameter of the canaliculus is 0.5 mm; however, it can be stretched to up to three times its normal diameter.

The lacrimal canaliculi are lined by stratified squamous epithelium.

13 **A** = True   **B** = True   **C** = False   **D** = False   **E** = False   **F** = False

The lacrimal sac is 12 mm long and lined (as with the nasolacrimal duct) by two layers of columnar epithelium, the deeper being slightly flatter. It is related medially to the anterior ethmoidal air cells above and the middle meatus of the nose below. Anteriorly, the medial palpebral ligament is related to its upper half. With regards to the surgical approach to the lacrimal sac, care must be taken not to approach more than 3 mm medial to the medial canthus as the angular vein crosses the medial palpebral ligament approximately 8 mm medial to the medial canthus, and occasionally angular vein tributaries may also be found between the vein and the canthus.

The nasolacrimal duct is 18 mm long and passes downwards, backwards and laterally. It lies lateral to the middle meatus and makes an indentation into the medial wall of the maxillary sinus.

14 **A** = True   **B** = False   **C** = False   **D** = True   **E** = False

The eyeball lies superolaterally in the orbital cavity and anteriorly, so that one-third of the globe lies in front of an imaginary plane between the medial and lateral orbital margins. The globe consists of an anterior segment and a posterior segment. Its anteroposterior diameter is 24 mm and the axis passes through a point in between the optic disc and the fovea. It may be as high as 29 mm in myopes or as low as 20 mm in hypermetropes. The vertical diameter is 23 mm and is less than the horizontal diameter of 23.5 mm.

15 **A** = False   **B** = False   **C** = False   **D** = False   **E** = True

Corneal diameters are approximately 11.7 mm horizontally and 10.6 mm vertically. The cornea has a thickness of approximately 0.5–0.6 mm in its central portion and 1 mm peripherally. The radius of curvature of the anterior surfaces is 7.8 mm and the posterior surface 6.5 mm. The cornea is usually more curved in the vertical axis than in the horizontal axis. It is more curved in the central third portion and flatter peripherally. The refractive index of the cornea is 1.36 and the anterior surface is largely responsible for the power of refraction.

16 **A** = True   **B** = False   **C** = False   **D** = False   **E** = True

The epithelium is 50–60 μm thick and is 10% of the corneal thickness. It is made up of a stratified non-keratinized epithelium, five cell layers centrally and thickening to up to 12 cells at the limbus. It is made up of three layers: a flat superficial layer of approximately three cells thick, attached to each other by desmosomes, a second layer of polyhedral 'wing'-shaped cells, and a basal layer made up of a single layer of tall columnar cells interdigitating with one another and attached by desmosomes and hemidesmosomes to the underlying basement membrane. It is important to note that the cornea does not possess epithelial stem cells and regeneration depends on centripetal migration from the mitotic limbal stem cells.

Bowman's membrane is an acellular layer approximately 10 μm thick containing a matrix of collagen fibrils. Unlike the stroma, there are no fibroblasts in Bowman's membrane.

17 **A** = True   **B** = True   **C** = False   **D** = False   **E** = False

Descemet's membrane is regarded as the endothelial basement membrane. It is between 6 and 10 μm thick and increases in thickness throughout life. It has an anterior fibrillar layer and a posterior granular layer where the main growth occurs. At the limbus, Descemet's membrane appears to be continuous with the line of Schwalbe. The endothelial is a single layer of flat, hexagonal-shaped cells, interdigitating and also connected with one another by tight junctions. It continues beyond the limbus as endothelium lining the spaces of the angle.

18 **A** = True   **B** = True   **C** = False   **D** = True   **E** = True

The sclera (derived from the Greek word *skleros*, meaning 'hard') is 1 mm thick posteriorly, 0.6 mm thick at the equator and 0.3 mm behind the insertions of the recti (the thickness of the tendon and muscles result in the sclera being 0.6 mm thick at the insertion) and 0.8 mm thick near the corneoscleral limbus. The sclera is pierced by three groups of apertures: the posterior apertures around the optic nerve transmit the long and short ciliary nerves and vessels; the middle apertures located 4 mm behind the equator transmit the exiting vortex veins leaving from the choroid; the anterior apertures at the insertions of the recti transmit the anterior ciliary arteries (seven in total). The canal of Schlemm lies within the sclera deep to the limbus and is lined by endothelium.

19 **A** = False   **B** = True   **C** = True   **D** = False   **E** = True

The dense, hard, fibrous sclera is made up of collagen fibrils and irregularly arranged elastic fibres. The fibres are arranged circumferentialy around the optic disc and lamina cribrosa. Elsewhere, they are arranged in a net-like fashion with a circular arrangement anterior to the equator so that the recti interact at right-angles with the fibres at their insertion. The scleral collagen is mainly of type I and type III. Type IV collagen is found in the lamina cribrosa. The lamina cribrosa is the weakest part of the sclera. The sclera is relatively avascular and poorly innervated. The episclera, however is a highly vascular (receiving supply from the anterior ciliary arteries) zone of loose connective tissue that is thick anteriorly and becomes thinner towards the back of the eye.

20 A = False **B** = False **C** = True **D** = False **E** = False

The sclera is made up of approximately 68% water and remains opaque with values between 40% and 80%. It becomes transparent with levels less than 40% or greater than 80%. The inner layer of the sclera is formed by the lamina fusca formed by a thin irregular coating of melanocytes separating the sclera from the perichoroidal space. The long posterior ciliary arteries and nerves pierce the sclera nasally and temporarily at 3.6 mm and 3.9 mm from the optic nerve respectively. The optic nerve pierces the sclera 3 mm medial to the mid-line and 1 mm below the horizontal meridian of the globe.

The sclera decreases in thickness with age.

21 A = False **B** = False **C** = True **D** = False **E** = False

The ciliary body is continuous with the choroid and iris. It begins 1.5 mm behind the corneoscleral limbus in the vertical meridian only (at the scleral spur) and ends 7.5–8 mm behind the limbus on the temporal side and 6.5–7 mm behind the limbus on the nasal side. It is thus seen to be larger on the temporal side. The pars plicata has an anteroposterior length of 2 mm and the wider pars plana has an anteroposterior length of 3.5 mm (nasally) and 4 mm (temporally).

The pars plicata is made up of 70–80 folds forming the ciliary process.

22 A = True **B** = False **C** = False **D** = False **E** = True

Both the inner non-pigmented and outer pigmented ciliary epithelia are cuboidal in the young, however, with age the non-pigmented epithelial cells become columnar. The non-pigmented epithelia are attached to one another basolaterally by desmosomes and apicolaterally by zonulae occludentes ('tight junctions'), zonulae adherentes and gap junctions (2 nm clefts). The apicolateral tight junctions form an important component of the blood–aqueous barrier.

The greatest number of gap junctions in the ciliary epithelium are found between pigmented and non-pigmented cells. This allows them to function in close cooperation. Other junctions between pigmented and non-pigmented epithelial cells include desmosomes and 'modified focal zonulae adherentes' known as puncta adherentes.

23 **A** = True   **B** = True   **C** = False   **D** = True   **E** = False

The cuboidal pigmented ciliary epithelial cells are attached to one another by gap junctions, desmosomes and puncta adherentes. No zonulae occludentes are present and this is consistent with a lack of blood–aqueous barrier function here. Pigmented ciliary epithelial cells contain fewer mitochondria, less rough endoplasmic reticulum and less regular Golgi apparatus than the adjacent non-pigmented epithelial cells. Both layers of epithelial cells have a basement membrane. The outer layer basement membrane is continuous with the basement membrane of the outer retinal layers, and the inner layer basement membrane is continuous with the internal limiting membrane of the retina.

The capillary walls in the ciliary stroma are fenestrated.

24 **A** = False   **B** = True   **C** = False   **D** = False   **E** = True

The ciliary muscle fibres form the bulk of the ciliary body and are comprised of an outermost longitudinal (or meridional) component, a middle oblique (or radial) component and an inner circular or (sphincteric) part. The fibre bundles are surrounded by a sheath of fibroblasts (as opposed to collagen) and contain more abundant mitochondria and endoplasmic reticulum then normal smooth muscle. The Golgi apparatus is better developed. With age, dense collagen and granular material accumulates. Lipofuscin is seen to deposit after the age of 50.

The blood supply to the ciliary body is from the two long posterior ciliary arteries and the seven anterior ciliary arteries. These anastamose at the major arterial circle of the iris behind the root of the iris and in front of the radial portion of the ciliary muscle to supply a rich plexus to the ciliary processes. Recurrent branches of the long posterior ciliary arteries as well as 10–12 recurrent branches from the anterior ciliary arteries pass back to the choroid. The ciliary body also receives muscular branches from the major arterial circle.

Venous drainage is mainly by the vortex veins, but also to a small degree by the anterior ciliary vessels.

The ciliary body contains myelinated and non-myelinated nerve fibres carrying parasympathetic, sympathetic and sensory innervation. The ciliary muscle and ciliary body receive postganglionic parasympathetic innervation from the ciliary ganglion (via the Edinger–Westphal nucleus and oculomotor nerve). Sympathetic fibres from both the long ciliary nerves as well as accompanying fibres of the ciliary arteries are found mainly in the ciliary processes as well as the ciliary muscle. The role of these is uncertain. The role of the sensory innervation to the ciliary body is also uncertain.

25 **A** = True   **B** = False   **C** = False   **D** = True   **E** = False   **F** = False

See notes to Anatomy Question 27.

26 **A** = True   **B** = True   **C** = False   **D** = True   **E** = False

See notes to Anatomy Question 27.

27 **A** = True   **B** = False   **C** = True   **D** = True   **E** = False

The iris (after the Greek word meaning 'rainbow') has a diameter of 21 mm. It is divided by the colarette (the thickest part of the iris 2 mm from the inner pupillary margin) into the pupillary zone and a thinner peripheral ciliary zone. The iris is made up of three layers: an anterior surface, the stroma and sphincter pupillae muscle, and a posterior layer.

The anterior surface is made up of a dense compact and discontinuous arrangement of fibroblasts, melanocytes and collagen. Because of its density, this layer is distinct from the underlying stroma. The human iris does not contain an endothelial layer.

The *stroma* contains pigmented and non-pigmented cells including fibroblasts, melanocytes, clump cells, mast cells, macrophages, lymphocytes and extracellular matrix of loosely arranged collagen (diameter 40–50 nm, periodicity 50–60 nm), proteoglycans as well as blood vessels and nerves. The stroma does not contain elastic fibres. All arterial vessels, including capillaries, of the stroma have non-fenestrated endothelium. The *sphincter pupillae* is a flat ring of smooth muscle approximately 1 mm wide and is found at the pupillary zone around the circumference of the pupil. It is surrounded by collagen that also attaches it to the pupillary end of dilator pupillae.

The posterior layer is formed by the pigment epithelial cells and dilator pupillae muscle. The dilator pupillae is a thin layer of myoepithelium made up of smooth muscle and derived from the anterior pigment epithelium of the iris. It lies from the pupillary zone to the periphery of the iris. The pigment epithelium of the iris is made up of a bilayer of epithelial cells lying apex-to-apex behind the stroma. The anterior pigment epithelium is continuous with the pigment epithelium of the ciliary body and lies posterior to the stroma. The posterior epithelial cells are cuboidal and larger than the anterior epithelial cells. They become columnar when the pupil is dilated. They are more pigmented and contain a greater number of melanin granules.

28 **A** = True   **B** = True   **C** = True   **D** = False   **E** = False

The lens has an equatorial diameter of 10 mm and a thickness of 4–5 mm; however, the latter increases with accommodation. The anterior surface lies 3 mm from the posterior surface of the cornea. The lens is made up of a capsule, epithelium, lens fibres and zonules. The epithelium is a monolayer of cells just behind the capsule on the anterior surface of the lens.

29 **A** = True   **B** = False   **C** = True   **D** = True   **E** = True

The lens capsule is an homogeneous basement membrane structure. It is thickest just in front of and behind the equator and thinnest at the posterior pole (approximately 3 μm). The anterior capsule is up to three times thicker than the posterior capsule.

The epithelium of the lens is made up of a monolayer of cubodial cells.

The lens fibres are 12 mm long, U-shaped fibres tightly packed and attached to each other by interdigitating 'ball and socket' and 'tongue and groove' joints in the cortex and nucleus respectively. They form an innermost compact embryonic nucleus, followed by a foetal nucleus (with Y-shaped sutures), both of which remain constant in size after birth. Outside this lies the adult nucleus (increasing in size throughout life) and the cortex of young enucleated fibres.

Electron microscopy has shown that zonular fibres of the lens attach the capsule at and around the equator to the ciliary processes of the pars plicata as well as further posteriorly to a small aspect of the pars plana.

The radii of curvature of both anterior and posterior surfaces decrease with age.

30 **A** = True   **B** = True   **C** = False   **D** = True   **E** = False

The choroid is described as having four layers: (1) suprachoroid, (2) vessel layer, (3) choriocapillaris layer and (4) Bruch's membrane. It is made up of melanocytes, stroma mucinous fluid, vessels and nerves.

The arterial blood supply to the choroid is by the anterior as well as the long and short posterior ciliary arteries. The 20 or so short posterior ciliary arteries pierce the sclera mainly in the longitudinal plane more so on the temporal side within a 2.5 mm radius of the optic disc.

The choroid is innervated by the long and short ciliary nerves and fibres from the facial nerve. The long ciliary nerves supply sensory, sympathetic and some parasympathetic fibres to dilator pupillae. The short ciliary nerve also carries sensory, parasympathetic and some sympathetic fibres. Parasympathetic fibres in the choroid are mainly from the Edinger–Westphal nucleus and oculomotor nerve, however, vasomotor fibres from the facial nerve and pterygopalatine ganglion have also been found in the choroid.

The suprachoroidal space is the outer layer of the choroid and is approximately 30 μm thick. It is least seen at the macula due the density of vessels and nerves here passing from the sclera to choroid.

31 **A** = False   **B** = False   **C** = True   **D** = False   **E** = True

The choroid is at its thickest at the posterior pole (0.2–0.3 mm) becoming thinner peripherally (0.1 mm). Melanocytes are most densely found in the outer choroidal layers and decrease in density towards the inner layer. Except for the macula and adjacent area to the optic disc, the majority of the vessels seen in the choroid are veins. These choroidal veins mainly drain into the four vortex veins and the anterior ciliary veins. The choriocapillaris lies vitread to the layer of arteries and veins and sclerad to Bruch's membrane.

32 A = True **B** = False **C** = True **D** = False **E** = False

Continuous endothelial lining is found in the arteries, arterioles and veins of the choroid. The choriocapillaris has fenestrated endothelial cells surrounded by basement membrane and no smooth muscle. The stroma does not form a definite layer in the choroid but serves as a supporting structure of connective tissue surrounding the vessels (which take up the greatest volume of the choroid).

Bruch's membrane is the innermost layer of the choroid. It is said to have up to five layers and its inner basement membrane is separated from the retinal pigment epithelium cell membrane by a radiolucent zone. Bruch's membrane is thickest posteriorly near the disc (approximately 3 μm) and becomes thinner anteriorly (1 μm).

33 A = False **B** = True **C** = True **D** = True **E** = True

The foveola lies 3 mm (two disc margins) temporal to the temporal margin of the optic disc and 0.8 mm below the meridional plane of the centre of the optic disc. It is a depression containing cones only found in the centre of the fovea (1.5 mm or one disc in diameter). The retina is thinnest at the fovea (0.1 mm) and thickest at the perifoveal region (0.23 mm). It then gradually thins out towards the ora serrata (0.11 mm), stabilizing at the equator.

The foveola is a rod-free zone and rods remain absent within a 2.8 mm radius from the centre of the foveola.

34 A = True **B** = True **C** = False **D** = False **E** = False

The retina contains approximately 6.5 million cones, 100 000 of which are present in the fovea, and approximately 120 000 000 rods, most concentrated at the perifovea and outside the fovea and parafovea. Cones are most concentrated in number at the foveola (approximately 2500) and are packed perpendicular to the retinal surface. The inner segments are separated from each other by the supporting Müller cells forming the external limiting membrane.

One of the main differences between rods and cones is the fact that the outer membrane of the rod outer segment is discontinuous with the stack of 600–1000 discs enclosed. The outer membrane of the cone outer segment is continuous with the discs.

The photoreceptor is made up of an outer segment and an inner segment, an outer fibre separated from an inner fibre by a cell body and finally a spherule (rod) or pedicle (cone). The connecting stalk is an eccentrically placed 0.2 μm diameter modified cilium consisting of nine pairs of microtubules with no central pair.

35 **A** = True   **B** = False   **C** = True   **D** = False   **E** = False

The inner segment of the photoreceptor consists of an outer portion named the 'ellipsoid', rich in mitochondria and an inner portion, the 'myoid', rich in components for protein synthesis such as rough endoplasmic reticulum, ribosomes and Golgi apparatus.

Although not strictly 'layers', the retina is described as having ten layers (from vitreous to sclera): (1) internal limited membrane, (2) nerve fibre layer, (3) ganglion cell layer, (4) inner plexiform layer, (5) inner nuclear layer, (6) outer plexiform layer, (7) outer nuclear layer, (8) external limited membrane, (9) photoreceptor layer (rods and cones), and (10) retinal pigment epithelium.

The outer nuclear layer of the retina lies between the external limiting membrane and the outer plexiform layer and consists mainly of rod and cone cell bodies as well as inner and outer fibres. The external limiting membrane is a layer formed by the attachment of modified Müller cell membrane with rod and cone membranes and zonulae adherentes creating a dense visible line without gaps. The outer plexiform layer is formed by rod and cone inner fibres, synapses between photoreceptors, bipolar and horizontal cells and also by Müller cell processes. The outer plexiform layer lies between the inner and outer nuclear layers.

36 **A** = True   **B** = True   **C** = False   **D** = False   **E** = False   **F** = True

Ganglion cells do not exist at the fovea or optic disc. Müller cells extend from the external limiting lamina to the internal limiting lamina. They provide intercellular support. The internal limiting lamina is formed by end feet of the Müller cells and astrocytes and is a basement membrane covering the inner retinal surface with interactions with vitreous body collagen fibrils.

The central retinal vein lies temporal (or lateral) to the central retinal artery at the optic disc. The retinal arteries lie either vitread or sclerad to retinal veins beneath the internal limiting membrane in either the nerve fibre layer or the ganglion cell layer. They branch into arterioles and then capillaries that are distributed to all layers up to the inner nuclear layer.

37 **A** = True   **B** = True   **C** = True   **D** = False   **E** = True

Retinal capillaries are made of up of non-fenestrated endothelium, basement membrane and pericytes lining outside the endothelium.

Retinal pigment epithelial cells at the macula are taller and contain more melanin than in the retinal periphery. Xanthophyll pigment is also found at the macula in the outer plexiform layer (Henle's fibre layer) and these phenomena probably account for the darker appearance of the macula.

The basement membrane of the retinal pigment epithelium is continuous with that of the ciliary pigment epithelium and stops at the optic disc.

The retinal pigment epithelial cells are attached to each other at their apicolateral surfaces by zonulae occludentes and zonulae adherentes, forming a complex that encircles all apicolateral surfaces playing an important role in the blood–retinal barrier. They are attached to each other at their basolateral surfaces by desmosome-like attachments. Desmosomes (maculae adherentes) appear at intervals on the lateral surfaces of adjacent cells and form point attachments. They may be identified by their characteristic electron-dense intercellular plates and tonofilaments passing into the retinal pigment epithelium cytoplasm.

Retinal arteries are two-thirds to three-quarters the diameter of retinal veins.

38 A = True **B** = True **C** = True **D** = True **E** = True

The four rectus muscles arise from the tendinous ring (of Zinn). They are each approximately 40 mm in length. The superior rectus has the longest muscle length, followed by the medial rectus then the lateral rectus and lastly, the inferior rectus. They run close to the orbital wall and beyond the equator form tendons that insert into the sclera. The lateral rectus has the longest tendon length (8.8 mm) followed by the superior rectus (5.8 mm) then the inferior rectus (5.5 mm) and lastly the medial rectus (3.7 mm). The medial rectus inserts into the sclera closest to the limbus (5.5 mm), followed by the inferior rectus (6.5 mm) then the lateral rectus (6.9 mm) and last, the superior rectus (7.7 mm).

39 A = True **B** = False **C** = False **D** = True **E** = False

The superior oblique arises above and medial to the optic canal and after a muscle length of approximately 32 mm becomes a tendon. One centimetre further, it hooks around the trochlea and turns back at an angle of 54° to the sagittal plane to insert into the sclera after passing beneath the superior rectus.

The inferior oblique arises from the orbital plate at the maxilla behind the lower orbital margin and lateral to the nasolacrimal duct. It passes back at an angle of 51° to the sagittal plane, beneath the inferior rectus to insert into the sclera.

As a simple rule: the obliques pass beneath the recti.

A thickening of the inferior rectus sheath passes forward to insert into the lower lid and is known as the lower lid retractor.

The medial rectus is innervated by the inferior division of the oculomotor nerve.

40 **A** = False   **B** = True   **C** = True   **D** = False   **E** = False

The lacrimal nerve and artery lie above the lateral rectus. The ophthalmic artery passes below the superior rectus to either cross over (or under) the optic nerve. It then passes medial to the globe above the medial rectus.

    The superior division of the oculomotor nerve pierces (and innervates) the superior rectus before terminating in levator. The trochlea nerve emerges from the superior orbital fissure within the common tendinous ring and enters the superior surface of the superior oblique muscle soon after, fairly close to the muscle origin (not insertion).

41 **A** = True   **B** = True   **C** = True   **D** = False   **E** = False   **F** = True

The ophthalmic artery arises from the internal carotid artery after it passes from the cavernous sinus and lies medial to the anterior clinoid process and below the optic nerve. It lies in the subarachnoid space and passes laterally and forwards within the dural sheath throughout its course in the optic canal. Early on in the orbital cavity it lies medial to the ciliary ganglion before passing over the optic nerve (15% pass under) towards the medial wall of the orbit. It then passes forwards and divides terminally into the dorsal nasal artery and the supratrochlear artery.

42 **A** = True   **B** = True   **C** = True   **D** = False   **E** = True

The central retinal artery arises from the ophthalmic artery inferolaterally to the optic nerve. It pierces the dural sheath 12.5 mm from the eyeball and crosses the subarachnoid space below the optic nerve before piercing the inferomedial surface of the optic nerve.

    The lacrimal artery usually arises once the ophthalmic artery leaves the optic canal. It runs with the lacrimal nerve on the upper border of the lateral rectus.

    The anterior and posterior ethmoidal arteries are branches of the ophthalmic artery. The anterior ethmoidal artery (larger than the posterior ethmoidal artery) passes through the anterior ethmoidal canal, anterior cranial fossa and cribriform plate before passing beneath the nasal bone to emerge between the bone and the lateral nasal cartilage and supply an area of the tip of the nose. It supplies the frontal sinus and anterior and medial ethmoidal sinuses. Whilst in the anterior fossa it also gives off a meningeal branch to supply the dura of the anterior cranial fossa.

    The anterior ciliary arteries arise from the muscular branches of the ophthalmic artery. Except for the lateral rectus, which gives rise to one anterior ciliary artery, each rectus muscle gives rise to two anterior ciliary arteries.

43 **A** = True   **B** = True   **C** = True   **D** = False   **E** = False

The cavernous sinus receives blood from the superior and inferior ophthalmic veins, the central retinal vein, the superficial middle cerebral vein, the inferior cerebral veins and the sphenoparietal sinus. It drains to the transverse sinus via the superior petrosal sinus, the internal jugular vein via the inferior petrosal sinus and the pterygoid plexus via emissary veins passing through foramen ovale. By communication with the superior ophthalmic vein it may also drain to the facial vein.

44 **A** = True   **B** = False   **C** = True   **D** = True   **E** = False

The cavernous sinus extends between the superior orbital fissure and the apex of the petrous temporal bone. It is approximately 2 cm long and 1 cm wide and lies beside the body of the sphenoid bone. It lies lateral to the sphenoidal sinus and hypophysis cerebri and medial to the uncus. The trigeminal cave and ganglion lie inferoposterior to the cavernous sinus.

The superior ophthalmic vein receives blood from the central retinal vein. The central retinal vein leaves the optic nerve 10 mm from the eyeball and lies in the subarachnoid space before either joining the superior ophthalmic vein or the cavernous sinus directly.

The inferior ophthalmic vein passes back in the orbital cavity and may be found lying above the inferior rectus. It communicates via the inferior orbital fissure with the pterygoid venous plexus and often communicates with the cavernous sinus via the superior orbital fissure.

45 **A** = True   **B** = True   **C** = False   **D** = True   **E** = False   **F** = False

The optic nerve is made up of an intraocular part (10 mm), a tortuous intraorbital part (25–30 mm) and an intracanalicular part (5 mm) and an intracranial part (10 mm). The optic chiasma measures 8 mm anteroposteriorly, 12 mm wide and 4 mm thick. It usually lies 'post-fixed' 10 mm directly above the dorsum sellae (although may lie 'pre-fixed' directly above the sella turcica itself).

Nasal retinal fibres decussate at the optic chiasma. The fibres corresponding to the inferonasal retina are related to the anterior portion of the optic chiasma. Superonasal retinal fibres are related to the posterior portion of the optic chiasma.

The arterial blood supply to the intracranial portion of the optic nerve is by its pial plexus which is supplied by the superior hypophyseal artery (from the internal carotid artery) and the ophthalmic artery. It also receives a few branches from the anterior cerebral artery.

The optic tract fibres correspond to the ipsilateral temporal retina and contralateral nasal retina. These relate to the contralateral field. Inferior retinal fibres correspond to lateral fibres of the optic tract and superior retinal fibres correspond to medial fibres of the optic tract. Macular fibres lie centrally and towards the lateral geniculate nucleus adopt a more dorsolateral position in cross-section.

46 A = True   **B** = False   **C** = False   **D** = True   **E** = True

Fibres of the ipsilateral temporal retina synapse in layers 2, 3 and 5 of the lateral geniculate nucleus and fibres of the contralateral nasal retina synapse in layers 1, 4 and 6. Superior retinal fibres correspond to the ventromedial portion of the lateral geniculate nucleus and inferior retinal fibres correspond to the dorsolateral portion. Macular fibres correspond to a wedge-like area in the most dorsal portion of the lateral geniculate nucleus.

The loop of Meyer refers to the fibres of the optic radiation (corresponding to the inferior retinal quadrants) that swing out furthest before turning medially to reach the lower lip of the calcarine sulcus. As these fibres bend out, they are related inferolaterally to the anterior tip of the temporal horn of the lateral ventricle. It explains the superior quadrantanopia defect seen in temporal lobe lesions.

47 A = True   **B** = False   **C** = True   **D** = True   **E** = False   **F** = True

The third ventricle is a slit-like cavity whose lateral walls are formed by the thalamus. It receives a communication from the two lateral ventricles via the interventricular foramina (of Monro) and continues caudally through the mid-brain as the narrow aqueduct of Sylvius, eventually arriving at the fourth ventricle.

The fourth ventricle lies in the pons and upper medulla. It has a mid-line slit-like aperture (the foramen of Magendie) and two lateral apertures that open anteriorly (foramina of Luschka). These form the only ports of exit of cerebrospinal fluid from the ventricles.

The lateral ventricle is described as a C-shaped cavity lying in the cerebral hemisphere. It is lined by ependymal cells and is made up of an anterior, posterior and inferior horn as well as a body. The anterior horn is enclosed by its roof, the fibres of the corpus callosum.

Inferomedially, a small aperture, the interventricular foramen of Monro communicates the lateral ventricle with the third ventricle. Behind the level of this foramen lies the body of the lateral ventricle. Its floor is the thalamus and body of the caudate nucleus. Its roof is the corpus callosum. The posterior horn lies above the collateral sulcus. Its medial wall is made up above by the fibres of forceps major (splenium of corpus callosum) and below by the calcar avis (formed by the calcarine sulcus). The optic radiations lie against the lateral wall of the posterior horn of the lateral ventricle.

48 A = False   **B** = False   **C** = False   **D** = False   **E** = True

The oculomotor nerve emerges from the mid-brain medial to the cerebral peduncles. Each oculomotor complex innervates the ipsilateral medial rectus, inferior rectus and inferior oblique as well as the contralateral superior rectus and levators on both sides.

The ciliary ganglion is a peripheral ganglion lying between the optic nerve and the lateral rectus. It is usually found lateral to the ophthalmic artery. It receives preganglionic parasympathetic fibres from the nerve to the inferior oblique (a branch of the oculomotor nerve).

The oculomotor nerve does not supply the lacrimal gland and therefore section does not result in increased lacrimation.

49 **A** = True   **B** = True   **C** = False   **D** = True   **E** = True   **F** = False

The trochlear nerve is the thinnest cranial nerve. It enters the orbital cavity through the superior orbital fissure outside the common tendinous ring medial to the frontal nerve. In the orbital cavity the trochlea nerve passes medially above levator to pierce the superior oblique. It is the only cranial nerve to emerge from the brainstem from its dorsal aspect.

The IV nucleus lies in the floor of the aqueduct (of Sylvius) in the mid-brain and also medial to the medial longitudinal fasciculus. Connections include the rostral interstitial nucleus of the medial longitudinal fasciculus and the medial longitudinal fasciculus itself, connecting it to the III, VI and VIII nuclei. Fibres from the IV nucleus decussate as they pass posteriorly before emerging from the dorsal aspect of the mid-brain. The IV nucleus innervates the contralateral superior oblique.

50 **A** = True   **B** = True   **C** = True   **D** = True   **E** = False   **F** = False

Sensory fibres of the trigeminal nerve carrying pain and temperature sensation are somatotopically organized in the spinal tract. Fibres from the ophthalmic division lie ventrolaterally, followed by those of the maxillary division and finally the fibres from the mandibular division lie dorsomedially. General visceral afferents from the glossophar-yngeal, vagus and facial nerves form a column adjacent and dorsal to the spinal tract.

The frontal nerve is the largest branch of the ophthalmic division followed by the intermediate sized nasociliary nerve and lastly the smallest branch, the lacrimal nerve.

Stimulation of the ophthalmic division of the trigeminal nerve in ophthalmic surgery may lead to the oculocardiac reflex and an afferent vagal output resulting in severe bradycardia or even asystole. Sensory innervation to the skin of the face is carried by the trigeminal nerve. A useful mnemonic is <u>LaSSIE IZZ A Big Mongrel</u>:

1 <u>The ophthalmic division</u>: <u>L</u>acrimal nerve, <u>s</u>upraorbital nerve, <u>s</u>upratrochlear nerve, <u>i</u>nfratrochlear nerve and <u>e</u>xternal nasal nerve.
2 <u>The maxillary division</u>: The <u>i</u>nfraorbital nerve, the <u>z</u>ygomaticofacial nerve, <u>z</u>ygomati-cotemporal nerve.
3 <u>The mandibular division</u>: <u>A</u>uriculotemporal nerve, <u>b</u>uccal nerve and <u>m</u>ental nerve.

The auriculotemporal nerve arises from the posterior division, splits briefly to enclose the middle meningeal artery and then passes back to the neck of the mandible. The auricular part of the auriculotemporal nerve innervates the skin of the tragus, the upper part of the pinna, the external ear canal and the outer surface of the tympanic mem-brane. The temporal part of the auriculotemporal nerve supplies the skin of the temple.

Although the auriculotemporal nerve carries hitch-hiking postganglionic secretomotor fibres from the otic ganglion to the parotid gland, it does not innervate the parotid fascia enclosing the gland. This is innervated by the great auricular nerve (C2).

51 **A** = False   **B** = True   **C** = True   **D** = True   **E** = False

The sixth nucleus innervates the ipsilateral lateral rectus. The abducent nerve emerges from the brainstem at the lower border of the pons. After arching over the ridge of the petrous temporal bone and passing through Dorello's canal it passes through the cavernous sinus lying lateral to and running parallel with the internal carotid artery. Here it briefly receives sympathetic fibres from the internal carotid sympathetic plexus which then leave to join the ophthalmic division of the trigeminal nerve. This would explain how the long ciliary nerves of the nasociliary nerve (Va) supply sympathetic innervation to the eye.

52 **A** = False   **B** = True   **C** = True   **D** = True   **E** = True   **F** = True

The facial nerve is made up of a motor component and a sensory component, the nervus intermedius (which also carries preganglionic parasympathetic efferent fibres). The greater petrosal nerve, which essentially is a branch of the nervus intermedius portion, leaves the main facial nerve at the geniculate ganglion. It passes through the petrous temporal bone, beneath the temporal lobe and the underlying dura of the middle cranial fossa under the trigeminal ganglion until it is joined by the deep petrosal nerve (sympathetic fibres from the internal carotid plexus), now called the nerve of the pterygoid canal.

Passing through the pterygoid canal it reaches the pterygopalatine fossa where the preganglionic parasympathetic fibres synapse at the pterygopalatine ganglion. The postganglionic parasympathetic fibres are thought to either hitch-hike along the maxillary and the zygomatic nerve to reach the lacrimal nerve or enter via the inferior orbital fissure in what is known as the retro-orbital plexus to supply secretomotor innervation to the lacrimal gland. The special sensory taste fibres of the greater petrosal nerve as well as some sympathetic fibres pass straight through the pterygopalatine ganglion and are distributed amongst the sensory nerves of the maxillary divison of the trigeminal nerve. It is by these that taste fibres are carried from the hard and soft palate.

The chorda tympani is a branch of the facial nerve, once again, essentially part of the nervus intermedius. It receives taste innervation (not somatic sensation) from the anterior two-thirds of the tongue and supplies preganglionic parasympathetic secreto-motor fibres to the the submandibular ganglion. Motor branches of the facial nerve include (in order): nerve to stapedius, the posterior auricular nerve (to the occipital belly of occipitofrontalis) given off along with the muscular nerve to the posterior belly of digastric soon after emerging from the stylomastoid foramen, and finally, the temporal, zygomatic, buccal, mandibular and cervical divisions arising beyond the pes anserinus in the parotid gland.

53 **A** = False   **B** = False   **C** = True   **D** = False   **E** = False   **F** = False

The pterygomandibular raphé consists of interdigitating fibres of buccinator and superior constrictor. It attaches from the pterygoid hamulus down to the mandible just above and behind the posterior end of the mylohyoid line.

Buccinator (the trumpeter's muscle) helps in returning food from the cheek to between the teeth. It is accessory to the muscles of mastication and is innervated by the facial nerve.

The arterial supply to the scalp is by the external carotid artery (occipital, posterior auricular and superficial temporal arteries) and the internal carotid artery (supraorbital and supratrochlear). They anastomose most at the junction between the forehead and the temple. The superficial temporal artery is a terminal branch of the external carotid artery. It passes up behind the temporomandibular joint, passing in front of the tragus and finally branches out supplying skin over the temporalis fascia. A deep branch, the middle temporal artery runs alongside the squamous part of the temporal bone deep to the temporalis muscle.

The scalp is made up of five layers (SCALP): skin, connective tissue, aponeurosis, loose areolar tissue and the pericranium. The anastomosing arteries lie in the connective tissue and are seen to bleed heavily in scalp lacerations due to the fact that whilst embedded in dense connective tissue they are held open.

Temporalis inserts into the mandible from the mandibular notch to the coronary process. Its upper fibres elevate the jaw and its posterior fibres retract the jaw. Medial pterygoid has a deep head arising from the medial side of the lateral pterygoid plate and fossa, and a superficial head arising from the tuberosity of the maxilla and pyramidal process of the palatine bone. It inserts into the medial aspect of the angle of the mandible and acts to elevate, protract and laterally displace the mandible to the opposite side (for chewing). Temporalis is the only muscle to retract the mandible.

54 **A** = False   **B** = True   **C** = True   **D** = True   **E** = False

The thyroid gland ('shield-like') is made up of two lobes and an isthmus lying in front of the second third and fourth tracheal rings. The gland is completely enclosed in pretracheal fascia, thus accounting for the gland moving up and down with the larynx during swallowing.

The arterial supply to the thyroid gland is by the superior and inferior thyroid arteries. The superior thyroid artery is the first branch of the anterior aspect of the external carotid artery and descends in front of the external laryngeal nerve after giving off its superior laryngeal branch towards the apex of each lobe.

The inferior thyroid artery is a branch of the thyrocervical trunk (a branch of the first part of the subclavian artery) and the left rises in front of the left recurrent laryngeal nerve (occasionally the right runs behind the right recurrent laryngeal nerve) towards the lower pole of each gland. The inferior thyroid artery is the sole arterial blood supply to the upper and lower parathyroid glands.

The venous drainage of the thyroid gland is by the superior, middle and inferior thyroid veins. The superior thyroid vein usually drains directly into the internal jugular vein, however occasionally via the facial vein. The middle thyroid vein drains directly into the internal jugular vein. The inferior thyroid vein drains into the brachiocephalic vein (usually the left).

55 **A** = True **B** = True **C** = False **D** = False **E** = False **F** = False **G** = True
   H = True

The cervical sympathetic trunk carries preganglionic sympathetic fibres to synapse at the superior middle and inferior cervical ganglia. It continues up from the thorax and passes anterior to the neck of the first rib. At this point it lies medial to the supreme intercostal vein (which lies medial to the superior intercostal artery followed by the first thoracic nerve) ('SVAT'). The inferior cervical ganglion lies here anterior to the neck of the first rib behind the start of the vertebral artery.

Continuing up, the cervical sympathetic trunk runs medial to the vertebral artery in the root of the neck and lies in front of the prevertebral fascia. The middle cervical ganglion arises at the level of C6 vertebra medial to the carotid tubercle (of Chassaignac) and anterior to the vertebral artery.

Note that the vertebral artery enters the transverse foramen at the level of C6 vertebra. In its course it lies in front of the inferior cervical ganglion and behind the middle cervical ganglion. The cervical trunk runs up behind the carotid sheath and medial to the vagus nerve. It terminates at the superior cervical ganglion anterior to the lateral mass of the atlas and axis. Section of the cervical sympathetic trunk results in a preganglionic Horner's syndrome with ipsilateral miosis, ptosis, anhydrosis of the face and enophthalmos.

56 **A** = True **B** = True **C** = False **D** = True **E** = True

The superior cervical ganglion supplies postganglionic fibres to the internal and external carotid arteries, their branches the pterygopalatine ganglion, the eye (internal carotid plexus), the pharyngeal plexus and the submandibular and otic ganglia (external carotid plexus). It also distributes fibres to C1–4 of the cervical plexus as well as fibres to the cardiac plexus.

The middle cervical ganglion supplies fibres to the subclavian artery and its branches, the inferior thyroid artery and thus to the trachea, lower larynx and upper oesophagus. It also distributes fibres to C5 and 6 of the cervical plexus (brachial plexus) and the cardiac plexus.

The inferior cervical ganglion supplies fibres to the vertebral artery and its branches (not the organs it supplies), C7 and 8 of the cervical plexus (brachial plexus) and to the cardiac plexus. All three cervical ganglia supply fibres to the cardiac plexus.

It is seen that the middle and inferior cervical ganglia supply sympathetic fibres to the upper limb (and therefore the hand). They receive preganglionic fibres from T1–6, however the majority of fibres from T1 go to the superior cervical ganglion.

In 'cervical sympathectomy' for excessive sweating of the hands, the second and third thoracic ganglia are removed, thus interrupting the fibres of T2–6 reaching the middle and inferior cervical ganglia. Fibres of T1 are able to pass via the first thoracic ganglion (or more often the stellate ganglion) to reach the superior cervical ganglion uninterrupted, thereby avoiding a Horner's syndrome.

57 **A** = False **B** = False **C** = True **D** = True **E** = True **F** = False **G** = False

The parotid gland and masseter lie in the parotid region. The facial artery (a branch of the anteromedial surface of the external carotid artery) emerges at the lower border of the mandible, crossing the bone anterior to masseter where it is palpable. The parotid gland is mainly a serous gland surrounded by a tough fibrous capsule derived from the investing layer of deep cervical fascia.

From the anteromedial surface of the parotid gland emerge the five branches of the facial nerve. Deep to this emerges the parotid duct and deep to this lies the retromandibular vein and the terminal branches of the external carotid artery (the maxillary artery and the superficial temporal artery). The preauricular lymph nodes lie deep as well as superficial to the parotid capsule and also exist within the parotid gland itself.

The parotid duct is 5 cm long and runs forward over the surface of masseter, turning inwards at its anterior border to pierce buccinator. It runs a very short course forward again, deep to the mucous membrane of the cheek (creating a non-return valve flap) before piercing the mucous membrane opposite the second upper molar tooth.

The parotid gland receives parasympathetic secretomotor fibres from the IX (glossopharyngeal) nerve by way of the lesser petrosal nerve. The preganglionic fibres synapse at the otic ganglion. Postganglionic fibres hitch-hike along the auriculotemporal nerve to reach the parotid gland.

58 **A** = False **B** = True **C** = False **D** = True **E** = True

See notes to Anatomy Question 60.

59 **A** = True **B** = False **C** = False **D** = False **E** = True

See notes to Anatomy Question 60.

60 **A** = True **B** = True **C** = True **D** = True **E** = True

The circle of Willis is formed by the internal carotid and basilar arteries only. The anterior cerebral artery arises from the internal carotid artery at the perforated substance and passes forward above the optic nerve. It communicates with the opposite side by the anterior communicating artery and from then on runs around the corpus callosum in the longitudinal fissure. The anterior cerebral artery supplies the corpus callosum, the medial surface of hemisphere as far back as the parieto-occipital sulcus, septum pellucidum, the anterior part of the putamen, the head of the caudate nucleus, the orbital surface of the frontal lobe (including the olfactory lobe) part of the chiasma and the intracranial portion of the optic nerve.

The anterior communicating artery is approximately 4 mm in length and lies anterosuperior to the optic chiasma. It connects the two anterior cerebral arteries in the longitudinal fissure. Its branches supply the optic chiasma, lamina terminalis and the hypothalamus. The optic chiasma receives blood from a pial plexus whose main supply are the superior hypophyseal branches of the internal carotid artery, the internal carotid artery itself, the anterior cerebral artery, the anterior communicating artery and the middle cerebral and posterior communicating arteries ('providing a few twigs') to its inferior surface.

The middle cerebral artery is the largest branch of the internal carotid artery. It runs laterally into the lateral sulcus before dividing into branches on the insula. The middle cerebral artery supplies the lateral aspect of the hemisphere except for a strip at the upper border supplied by the anterior cerebral artery and a strip at the lower border supplied by the posterior cerebral artery. It gives off striate arteries that pass at the base of the external capsule and supply the caudate and lentiform nuclei. It also supplies a few small branches to the optic chiasma, anterior optic tract and optic radiations. It contributes to the supply of the macula portion of the visual cortex by anastomosing with calcarine branches of the posterior cerebral artery. This gives rise to the phenomenon of 'macula sparing' with occlusion of the posterior cerebral artery causing a contralateral hemianopia and intact macula. Occlusion of the middle cerebral artery results in complete contralateral hemiplegia (including an upper motor neurone facial weakness affecting the contralateral lower face only), hemianaesthesia and aphasia (if the lesion affects the dominant hemisphere).

The posterior cerebral artery is a branch of the basilar artery and is formed by its bifurcation at the upper border of the pons. It passes around the inferior border of the cerebral peduncle and runs below the optic tract and above and parallel to the superior cerebellar artery. It passes above the tentorium cerebelli to supply the inferior surfaces of the temporal and occipital lobes. It supplies the posteromedial aspect of the lateral geniculate nucleus, the posterior two-thirds of the optic radiation and almost all of the visual cortex except for an anastomosis with the middle cerebral artery over the macular area at the occipital pole. Occlusion of the posterior cerebral artery produces a contralateral homonymous hemianopia, possibly with macula sparing and hemianaesthesia (posterior limb of internal capsule).

The posterior communicating artery arises from the internal carotid artery and runs back parallel with and above the oculomotor nerve to anastomose with the posterior cerebral artery. Its branches pierce the posterior perforated substance to supply the thalamus and the posterior limb of the internal capsule. It also supplies the anterior third of the optic tract (with the anterior choroidal artery supplying the posterior two-thirds) and gives a few small branches to the optic chiasma.

The basilar artery is formed at the lower border of the pons by the junction of the right and left vertebral arteries and bifurcates at the upper border of the pons into the right and left posterior cerebral arteries. It gives off pontine arteries to the pons, a labyrinthine artery to the internal ear, the anterior inferior cerebellar artery supplying the anterolateral area of the inferior surface of the cerebellum and inferolateral portion of the pons, the superior cerebellar arteries supplying the superior cerebellar surface and the pons, and finally the posterior cerebral arteries.

The pons is mainly supplied by the pontine branches of the basilar artery and occlusion of the basilar artery may affect bilateral motor pathways causing bilateral paralysis as well as other more common bulbar signs. The arterial supply to the optic tract is by branches from the anterior choroidal and posterior communicating arteries. The optic radiation is supplied by the anterior choroidal artery (anteriorly) and posterior cerebral artery (posteriorly) as well as deep branches from the middle cerebral artery.

PHYSIOLOGY
Questions

General Physiology

Cardiovascular

1 With regard to blood flow and blood vessels,

    A cardiac output can be determined using Fick's principle
    B velocity of blood flow through a vessel is proportional to the cross-sectional area
    C all capillaries are open under normal conditions at rest
    D haemaglobin concentration is not required in order to calculate cardiac output
    E the velocity of blood flow through capillaries is approximately 0.3 mm/s
    F blood flow is more likely to be turbulent in anaemia than when haemaglobin levels are normal
    G coronary blood flow is 10% of cardiac output

2 Which of the following statements about autoregulation are true?

    A Coronary blood flow is directly related to systolic blood pressure.
    B Skeletal muscle blood flow in exercise is increased mainly by sympathetic vasodilation.
    C Renal blood flow is directly related to mean blood pressure.
    D Pulmonary vasculature undergoes vasoconstriction in response to a rise in blood pressure.
    E Hypoxia causes vasoconstriction in pulmonary blood vessels.
    F A rise in local temperature causes vasodilation.

3 Regarding capillary exchange,

    A 5% of plasma flow is filtered by capillaries into the interstitial space
    B 30% of ultrafiltrate re-enters blood via lymph
    C capillary permeability to proteins is greatest in the liver
    D red blood cells increase in size as they pass through capillaries
    E haematocrit of blood decreases as it passes through capillaries
    F the haemoglobin dissociation curve shifts to the right as blood passes through a capillary

4 Baroreceptors

A are all in the arterial circulation
B stimulate vasoconstrictor activity through increased baroreceptor output
C reduce blood pressure by venodilation
D are found in cerebral arteries
E are found in retinal arteries

5 Which of the following statements concerning neural and hormonal control of blood flow are true?

A Vasodilation in genital organs is due β_2-adrenergic stimulation.
B Adrenaline is a vasoconstrictor in both low and high concentrations.
C Antidiuretic hormone (ADH) causes significant vasoconstriction *in vivo*.
D Pain results in a rise in blood pressure.
E Inspiration causes a rise in blood pressure.

6 Regarding blood pressure,

A mean pulmonary artery pressure is 10 mmHg
B pulse pressure is proportional to total peripheral resistance
C pulmonary hypertension occurs when living at high altitude
D the use of an inflatable cuff is a direct method of measuring blood pressure
E mean arterial blood pressure in a young adult is 120 mmHg

7 In the cardiac cycle,

A end-diastolic ventricular volume is 70 ml
B ventricular filling at rest is mainly due to atrial contraction
C systole begins when the aortic valve opens
D coronary blood flow to the right ventricle takes place only in diastole
E the v-wave of the jugular venous pulse is due to the closure of the tricuspid valve

8 Ventricular end-diastolic volume is increased by

A lying supine
B increased total blood volume
C venous contraction
D cardiac tamponade
E tachycardia

9 In foetal circulation

    A oxygenated foetal placental blood has an oxygen saturation of 65%
    B oxygenated blood flows from the umbilical artery to the ductus venosus
    C the ductus arteriosus closes within 12 hours of birth
    D oxygen saturation of blood in the umbilical artery is approximately 65%
    E at birth ventilation is stimulated by a rise in P_{CO_2}
    F the haemoglobin-dissociation curve is shifted to the left

Respiratory

10 Which of the following statements regarding gas exchange are correct?

    A P_{O_2} in dry air at sea level is 21 kPa.
    B P_{O_2} in expired air is 6 kPa.
    C The percentage of CO_2 in expired air is 15%.
    D Alveolar P_{CO_2} is identical to mixed venous P_{CO_2}.
    E Alveolar P_{CO_2} and P_{O_2} are reduced at high altitudes.
    F Alveolar P_{H_2O} is 47 mmHg.

11 In gas exchange,

    A lung surfactant increases alveolar surface tension
    B dead space equals tidal volume plus alveolar volume
    C physiological dead space is usually less than actual anatomical dead space
    D at rest alveolar volume is 70% of tidal volume
    E alveolar ventilation is increased by rapid shallow breathing
    F physiological dead space is increased by pulmonary embolus
    G anatomical dead space is approximately 300 ml
    H dead space is calculated using the Bohr equation

12 With regard to the mechanics of respiration,

    A intrapleural pressure is positive in forced expiration
    B pulmonary compliance is the ratio of change in intrapulmonary pressure per unit of change in volume
    C pulmonary compliance is the reciprocal of elastance
    D pulmonary compliance is reduced in emphysema
    E surfactant is produced by type I alveolar epithelial cells
    F intrapleural pressure is recorded using an intraoesophageal balloon

13 When calculating respiratory volumes, the following are used

    A Residual volume is measured using a spirometer.
    B Vital capacity is the tidal volume plus the inspiratory reserve volume.
    C Residual volume is greater or equal to functional residual capacity.
    D Inspiratory reserve volume is approximately 3 L in an adult.
    E Functional residual capacity is approximately 3 L in an adult.

14 With regard to alveolar surface tension,

    A lung surfactant allows collapse of alveoli
    B alveolar surface tension has its largest effect on increasing pulmonary static compliance
    C the LaPlace relationship relates surface tension in a sphere as a product of pressure and radius
    D lung surfactant is reduced in heavy smoking
    E lung surfactant predominantly contains lecithinase

15 Which of the following statements about ventilation and perfusion are true?

    A Alveolar ventilation is greater in the apex than in the base of the lung when upright.
    B When supine, the pulmonary blood flow (per unit volume) increases from apex to base.
    C The ventilation:perfusion ratio decreases from apex to base when erect.
    D Transection of the spinal cord above the level of C3 is fatal.
    E Physiological dead space causes a low ventilation:perfusion ratio.

16 Regarding CO_2 binding transport and distribution,

    A CO_2 is more soluble than O_2 in blood.
    B oxyhaemoglobin binds CO_2 more readily than does deoxyhaemoglobin
    C H^+ diffuses easily across the blood–brain barrier
    D carotid body chemoreceptors respond primarily to changes in P_{CO_2}
    E 20% of CO_2 in blood is bound to haemoglobin

17 In oxygen transport, binding and distribution,

    A mixed venous blood is 50% saturated with oxygen
    B cyanosis cannot occur without tissue hypoxia
    C central chemoreceptors are stimulated mainly by hypoxia

D the oxygen dissociation curve is shifted to the left in stored blood
E the oxygen dissociation curve is shifted to the right by a fall in pH

Renal

18 In the kidneys,

A production of 1α-hydroxylase occurs
B the proximal convoluted tubule cells do not possess a brush border
C the distal convoluted tubule cells have a rich brush border
D the macula densa exists at the distal convoluted tubule
E the distal convoluted tubule is rich in mitochondria

19 Which of the following statements about renal circulation are true?

A Renal blood flow is 25% of cardiac output.
B Autoregulation of renal blood flow occurs mainly at the level of the renal artery.
C Autoregulation of renal blood flow remains constant with mean arterial blood pressure between 40 and 200 mmHg.
D Renal blood flow may be calculated using the Fick's principle.
E Para-aminohippuric acid (PAH) is filtered by the glomerulus and reabsorbed by the proximal convoluted tubule cells.
F 50% of PAH is filtered through the kidney in each circulation.

20 Which of the following are correct?

A The GFR (glomerular filtration rate) in a normal adult is proportional to body surface area.
B The GFR in each kidney is 125 ml/min.
C The GFR is increased in diabetes insipidus.
D Blood urea concentration is a test of glomerular function.
E GFR is 20% of renal plasma flow.
F Urine volume varies from 1% to 20% of glomerular filtrate in a day.
G The GFR rate is measured by inulin clearance.

21 With regard to tubular transport,

A glucose is reabsorbed by secondary transport only in the proximal convoluted tubule
B creatinine, uric acid, potassium and H^+ ions are actively secreted into renal tubules

C only the proximal convoluted tubule and the collecting ducts are permeable to urea

D Na^+K^+ ATPase pump is found on the apical membrane of the tubular cells

E penicillin is mainly excreted by filtration at the glomerulus

22 Which of the following statements about sodium balance are true?

A Sodium reabsorption in the kidneys occurs from the proximal convoluted tubule to the collecting ducts inclusive.

B Seventy per cent of sodium is filtered in the proximal convoluted tubule.

C Sodium reabsorption is reduced by carbonic anhydrase inhibitors.

D Loop diuretics inhibit the Na^+K^+ ATPase pump at the thick ascending loop of Henle.

E Aldosterone increases sodium reabsorption at the collecting ducts.

23 With regard to water balance, which of the following are true?

A A 70 kg man is made up of approximately 42 L of water.

B One-third of body water content is extracellular.

C Plasma volume is 5% of total body water.

D A 3% minimum increase in serum osmolality is required to increase the release of antidiuretic hormone (ADH).

E Alcohol inhibits ADH release.

24 In the renin–angiotensin system,

A renin is produced and stored as pro-renin in the juxtaglomerular cells

B angiotensin II acts directly on the kidney to reduce salt and water excretion

C renin converts angiotensin I to angiotensin II

D aldosterone is produced at the zona glomerulosa

E primary hyperaldosteronism results in hypernatraemia

Endocrinology

25 With regard to the thyroid gland,

A thyroid-stimulating hormone (TSH) secretion is increased in iodine deficiency

B thyroxine increases oxygen uptake by cells

C hypercholesterolaemia is seen in hypothyroidism

D iodide uptake is seen in the ciliary body of the eye

E the half-life of thyroxine is 6 days

26 Which of the following statements about the thyroid are true?

    A Ninety-nine per cent of circulating T4 is bound to protein.
    B Thyroid hormones alter cell function by cell membrane receptor signalling.
    C Cerebrospinal fluid protein levels are raised in hypothyroidism.
    D TSH secretion peaks at midnight.
    E Thyroid hormones directly inhibit both TSH release at the anterior pituitary and thyrotrophin-releasing hormone (TRH) release from the hypothalamus.
    F T4 is more active than T3.

27 Glucagon

    A has a half-life of 5–10 min
    B is destroyed in the liver
    C is produced in the A cells of the islets of Langerhans
    D has the same structure in all mammals
    E secretion is inhibited by high levels of insulin

28 Insulin

    A increases potassium release from cells
    B has a half-life of 10–30 min
    C increases glucose uptake in the brain
    D is a steroid
    E increases gluconeogenesis in the liver

29 Vasopressin or ADH

    A secretion is reduced by pain
    B is produced by the posterior pituitary
    C increases water permeability at the loop of Henle
    D release increases with a fall in plasma osmolality of over 3 mOsm/kg H_2O
    E causes glycogenolysis in the liver

30 With regard to the pituitary,

    A the anterior pituitary directly regulates output of the adrenal medulla
    B hypophysectomy reduces aldosterone release
    C ACTH is not a steroid hormone
    D hypertension as a result of excess growth hormone is due to increased heart size resulting in increased cardiac output
    E prolactin is made up of an α and β subunit

31 In calcium metabolism,

  A hypercalcaemia is caused due to hyperthyroidism
  B hypercalcaemia is caused due to thiazide diuretic therapy
  C hypocalcaemia is caused due to chronic renal failure
  D hypercalcaemia is caused due to acute pancreatitis
  E hypercalcaemia causes secondary hyperparathyroidism

32 Which of the following statements about calcium are true?

  A A 70 kg man contains over 1 kg of calcium.
  B Parathyroid hormone is produced by the chief cells of the parathyroid gland.
  C Calcitonin is produced by the parafollicular C cells of the parathyroid gland.
  D Parathyroid hormone stimulates increased vitamin D production.
  E Oestrogen receptors in bone inhibit bone osteoclast activity.

33 With regards to glucocorticoids,

  A glucocorticoids cause an increase in the glomerular filtration rate
  B aldosterone secretion is increased in phaeochromocytoma
  C increased levels of glucocorticoids are associated with eosinophilia
  D aldosterone receptors are intracellular
  E glucocorticoids in the circulation are mostly bound to transcortin
  F aldosterone in the circulation exists largely unbound to protein
  G aldosterone is a 21 carbon 18-hydroxycorticosteroid

34 Which of the following statements about catecholomines are true?

  A Dopamine, tyrosine and phenylalanine are precursors of adrenaline.
  B The half-life of adrenaline is approximately 2 min.
  C Adrenaline in the circulation causes an increase in both systolic and diastolic arterial blood pressure.
  D Metabolites of adrenaline and noradrenaline in urine include VMA and 5-HIAA.
  E Adrenalectomy results in reduced plasma levels of noradrenaline and adrenaline.

CNS

35 Cerebrospinal fluid

  A absorption is due to sodium transport
  B protein content is approximately 20–40 mg/l

C rate of production is approximately 20 ml/h
D volume is 150 ml
E is not produced in the aqueduct of Monro
F has a lower pH than plasma
G normal lumbar pressure is 20–25 cmCSF

36 Which of the following statements about the CNS are true?

A The anterior spinothalamic tract conveys (mainly) signals of touch.
B Dorsal columns carry signals of proprioception.
C In the dorsal column, sacral and lumbar fibres are medial to thoracic and cervical fibres.
D In the spinothalamic tract, sacral and lumbar fibres are more medial than thoracic and cervical fibres.
E The anterior corticospinal tract contains the majority of corticospinal fibres.
F Babinski's sign results from damage to the lateral corticospinal tract.

37 With regard to the tendon reflexes,

A the knee jerk is a monosynaptic reflex elicited by stimulation of quadriceps tendon organs
B the ankle jerk is a monosynaptic stretch reflex
C Golgi tendon organs are stimulated by passive stretch as well as active muscle contraction
D muscle spindle afferents synapse directly on to ipsilateral homonymous α-motor neurones
E muscles spindles are stimulated by contraction of extrafusal fibres

38 In the cerebellum,

A the flocculonodular lobe receives proprioceptive information from the body
B resting tremor is a feature in cerebellar lesions
C Purkinje cells are inhibitory
D cerebellar hemispheric lesions affect the contralateral side of the body
E spastic knee jerks are seen in cerebellar disease
F lesions of the lateral cerebellar hemisphere produces truncal ataxia

Ocular physiology

The tears

39 Which of the following statements about tears are correct?

A Tear fluid contains lactoferrin.
B Aqueous tear production remains relatively constant with age.
C Basal tear production is 1.2 ml/h.
D The mucin layer is made up of an inner tight glycocalyx produced by the corneal epithelial cells.
E Corneal goblet cells contribute to the mucin layer.

40 With regard to structures associated with tears,

A the precorneal tear film has a thickness of 10 μm
B the outer hydrophobic lipid layer is produced by the glands of Zeiss, glands of Moll and meibomian glands
C the aqueous layer is usually slightly hypertonic
D general anaesthesia reduces tear production
E the lacrimal gland is a tubuloacinar gland, comprising of mainly tubular cells

41 Regarding tears,

A lipid meibom has a higher melting temperature than skin sebaceous secretions
B contact lens wearing causes an abnormal tear film with faster and greater evaporation
C 85% of tears are drained by the lower canaliculus
D partial pressure of oxygen in tears with eyelids open is approximately 155 mmHg
E partial pressure of oxygen in tears with eyelids closed is approximately 55 mmHg

The eyelids

42 Which of the following statements about the eyelids are true?

A Cilia are replaced every two months.
B Orbicularis oculi is an example of a yoke muscle.
C Bell's phenomenon occurs during reflex blink closure of the eyelids.
D The chronaxie of the palpebral portion of orbicularis oculi is half that of the orbital portion.
E Spontaneous blinking may change in response to changes in visual acuity.

43 With regards to the eyelids,

    A the fast component of the corneal blink reflex is ipsilateral and disynaptic with a latency of 10–15 ms

    B oedema or haematoma commonly collects within and distends the pretarsal space

    C the glands of Zeiss are less numerous than the glands of Moll

    D the conjunctival epithelium largely consists of non-keratinized stratified columnar epithelium

    E Müller's muscle is a smooth muscle innervated by sympathetic nerves in both upper and lower eyelids

44 Regarding the eyelids, which of the following are true?

    A Myokymia or fibrillary twitching of the eyelids is associated with fatigue.

    B The skin layer of the eyelid is glabrous (hairless).

    C Cilia have a very high threshold for tactile sensation.

    D At photopic levels, blinking with a duration of up to 10 ms shows no discontinuity of visual perception.

    E The long, thin ducts of the sebaceous glands of Zeiss empty directly into ciliary follicles.

Cornea

45 Which of the following statements about the cornea are true?

    A During sleep, oxygen delivery to the cornea is via the bulbar conjunctiva.

    B Epithelial oedema reduces contrast sensitivity.

    C The periphery of the cornea is the most sensitive area of the eye.

    D Basal cells of the epithelium are laterally interdigitated to one another by zonulae adherens and gap junctions, and inferiorly attached to the basal lamina by hemidesmosomes.

    E Thickenings of Descemet's membrane (Hassall–Henle 'warts') are common in the corneal periphery.

46 With regard to the cornea,

    A up to 80% of normal corneal endothelial cells are hexagonal in shape

    B the cornea displays 'temperature reversal' in that its thickness is reduced with reduced surrounding temperature and returns to normal in normal temperature

    C transendothelial potential is 5 mV

D *in vivo* use of carbonic anhydrase inhibitors is associated with impaired 'endothelial pump' function and some corneal swelling

E stromal active sodium concentration is 134 mEq/l

47 In the cornea,

A normal corneal swelling pressure is 35 mmHg

B swelling pressure is influenced by positively charged glycosaminoglycans in the stroma

C evaporation once the eyes are open accounts for 5% of corneal thinning during the day

D in response to stromal wounding, stromal keratocytes are seen to hypertrophy and proliferate

E in response to penetrating stromal wounds, tensile strength reaches normal levels by six months

F the corneal stroma consists of 78% water

48 Which of the following statement about the cornea are correct?

A Immediate events after corneal abrasion include an increase in the hemidesmo-somal attachment of cells at the wound edge to the basement membrane.

B Immediate events after corneal abrasion include an increase in mitosis.

C Epithelial cell migration can be increased in the presence of cholera toxin.

D The transepithelial potential of the corneal epithelium is approximately −70 mV.

E Choride ions enter the corneal epithelial via the 'Cl⁻ current' of secondary active co-transport and diffuse passively out of tears.

F Installation of fluorescein dye is a reliable clinical test of whether the junctional complexes along the lateral walls of the superficial cells are intact.

49 With regard to the cornea,

A the cornea transmits radiation from 310 nm to a maximum of 900 nm

B corneal epithelium contains keratin

C turnover of the entire epithelium is within 7 days

D basal cells of the corneal epithelium form a single layer of columnar epithelium

E the collagen of the corneal stroma is mainly type I variety

50 Regarding the cornea, which of the following statements are true?

A The cornea possesses a vascular endothelium with a high metabolic activity.

B The cornea derives its energy largely from anaerobic metabolism.

C The posterior surface of the cornea provides the major refractive component of the eye.

D The superficial cell layer of the epithelium is covered with a thick layer of microvilli.

E The single layer of the corneal endothelial cells have a cell density of approximately 3500 cells per mm^2 at birth.

51 In the cornea,

A the cellular Bowman's layer consists of randomly arranged collagen fibrils

B Bowman's layer is one-fifth of the thickness of the corneal epithelium

C the basement membrane of the corneal epithelium consists mainly of type IV collagen in the centre

D the stroma forms 98% of the corneal thickness

E Descemet's membrane is 10–5 μm thick

52 Regarding the cornea,

A long-term contact lens use (greater than 6 years) is associated with endothelial cell loss

B the posterior layer of Descemet's membrane increases in thickness throughout life

C Descemet's membrane is extremely resistent to proteolytic enzymes

D the endothelium acts as a tight barrier between aqueous humour and stroma

E corneal innervation, with the presence of the neuropeptides substance P and calcitonin gene-related peptide (CGRP), exerts a trophic (nutritional) effect on corneal wound healing

53 Which of the following are true?

A Nerve axons that pass through the anterior stroma are usually unmyelinated with a covering layer of Schwann cells.

B Corneal stroma has a lamellar arrangement of collagen fibrils with a diameter of between 24 and 30 nm.

C Corneal sensitivity is influenced by pigmentation of the iris.

D The corneal epithelium has chemical receptors for high pH and hypertonic solutions.

E The cell size of normal corneal endothelial cells has a coefficient of variation (standard deviation of mean cell area/mean cell area) of 0.25.

F Endothelial cell density is the most useful indicator of normal endothelial stability.

Aqueous and ciliary epithelium

54 Which of the following statements are correct?

  A Aqueous production is 2.5 μl/s.
  B Pigmented ciliary epithelium is responsible for aqueous formation.
  C Ultrafiltration is responsible for up to 15% of aqueous formation.
  D Aqueous flow increases during sleep.
  E The corneal endothelium 'fluid pump' accounts for 15% of aqueous fluid production.

55 With regards to the aqueous,

  A the main pathway for aqueous outflow is via the trabecular meshwork and decreases with the Valsalva manoeuvre
  B uveoscleral outflow of aqueous is an energy-dependent active process
  C intraocular pressure in the general population has a normal Gaussian distribution with a mean of 16 mmHg
  D regular exercises are associated with long-term reduction in intraocular pressure
  E intraocular pressure increases with inspiration and decreases with expiration

56 Regarding the aqueous,

  A small quantities of complement are found in primary aqueous
  B the uveal layer of the trabecular meshwork poses greatest resistance to aqueous outflow
  C aqueous passing through the trabecular meshwork enters Schlemm's canal by bulk flow.
  D uveoscleral drainage of aqueous passes through the anterior chamber angle to reach the suprachoroidal space
  E pulsatile intraocular pressure is due to arterial blood flow into the central retinal artery

57 In the aqueous,

  A IgA is the only detectable immunoglobulin
  B protein concentration is less than 20 mg/100 ml
  C fibrinogen is present in significant amounts
  D insulin is present
  E active secretion by the ciliary epithelium is at a constant rate regardless of intraocular pressure

58 How many of the following statements about the aqueous are correct?

    A Glucose is transported by carrier mediator transport across the blood–aqueous barrier.

    B Intraocular pressure shows a diurnal variation with a peak occurring between 7 and 9 am.

    C Aqueous production increases with age.

    D Glucose concentration in aqueous is two-thirds that of plasma.

    E Partial pressure of oxygen in aqueous humour is between 30 and 40 mmHg.

59 With regard to the aqueous,

    A the blood–aqueous barrier is formed partly by the impermeable fenestrated iris vessels

    B the ciliary body plays a role in the secretion of hyaluronic acid into the vitreous

    C small lipid-soluble molecules are able to penetrate the blood–aqueous barrier

    D the anterior and posterior chamber are iso-osmolar with plasma

    E urea induces a greater fall in intraocular pressure than mannitol

60 Which of the following are correct?

    A The ciliary body is divided into a smooth pars plana anteriorly and a pars plicata posteriorly.

    B The basal aspect of the pigmented ciliary epithelium faces the ciliary stroma.

    C Gap junctions exist between pigmented and non-pigmented ciliary epithelial cells.

    D Tight junctions exist between the apices of the pigmented ciliary epithelial cells.

    E Capillaries of the ciliary body are similar to those in the liver sinusoids.

61 With regard to the ciliary epithelium and the aqueous,

    A non-pigmented ciliary epithelial cells are cuboidal

    B acetazolamide lowers the rate of the production of aqueous humour by up to 50%

    C ciliary channels exist between pigmented and non-pigmented ciliary epithelial cells

    D secondary aqueous is the result of primary aqueous reaching the anterior chamber

    E release of prostaglandins E and F in response to chemical or mechanical insult disrupts the blood–aqueous barrier

Pupil

62 Which of the following statements about the pupils are true?

A Pupil diameter range from 2 mm to a maximum of 6 mm.
B Pupil size is largest during adolescence.
C Simply physiological anisocoria is present in 10% of the population.
D In reaction to light, the latent period of the light reflex in bright light is 0.2 s.
E A supratentorial space-occupying lesion damaging the third nerve causes a tonic pupil.

63 Complications of pupillary dilation include

A blurred vision
B light sensitivity
C acute closed-angle glaucoma
D uveitis
E raised intraocular pressure

64 Pupil size is affected by

A iris pigment
B myopia (myopes have larger pupils than hypermetropes)
C distance of object of fixation
D sleep
E severe depression

65 Which of the following statements about pupillary defects are true?

A Dense lens opacities cause an afferent pupillary defect.
B Consensual light reflex is equally as strong as direct light reflex in the normal subject.
C An efferent pupillary defect describes a fixed dilated pupil.
D Adie's tonic pupils constrict less than the normal pupil to 0.1% pilocarpine.
E Argyll Robertson pupils are dilated, react well to accommodation, but react poorly to light.

66 Mydriasis

A can be induced by botulinum toxin
B is induced by atropine because it is a competitive antinicotinic antagonist of acetylcholine

C is induced by edrophonium

D and cycloplegia can be caused by phenylephrine

E can be caused by phenobarbitone

67 Which of the following statements about miosis are true?

A Histamine causes miosis.

B Morphine can cause miosis, both by its direct action on smooth muscle and via the central nervous system.

C Pilocarpine can abolish the pupillary light reflex for many hours after its miotic affect disappears.

D Rebound miosis is seen once the mydriatic affect of cocaine disappears.

E Thymoxamine causes miosis with no effect on the ciliary body.

68 With regard to Horner's and Pancoast's syndromes, which of the following are true?

A Congenital Horner's sydrome causes heterochromia iris.

B In unilateral Horner's, dilation lag and anisocoria are clearly present after 5 s during a sudden change from bright light to dark.

C Cocaine dilation is reduced in post-ganglionic Horner's pupils only.

D Based on the principle of denervation hypersensitivity, the adrenaline test is a reliable test in distinguishing pre- and post-ganglionic Horner's syndrome.

E Pancoast's syndrome is associated with failure of hydroxyamphetamine to dilate the affected pupil.

The lens

69 Which of the following statements about the lens are true?

A The lens plays a role in filtering infrared light.

B The capsule is mainly made up of type IV collagen.

C The capsule is synthesized by the lens epithelium and superficial lens fibres posteriorly.

D The lens is unique in its two-thirds protein content necessary for a high refractive index.

E The regular helical arrangement of lens proteins with small differences in refractive index plays a role in transparency.

70 In the lens,

   A the resting voltage is −70 mV
   B the potassium concentration is 125 mmol/l
   C 33% of the protein content is made up of water-soluble proteins
   D concentration of glutathione is 1000 times greater than that of the aqueous humour
   E glutathione concentrations are found to be raised in the presence of cataracts

71 With regard to the lens,

   A central lens epithelial cells are columnar
   B crystallins are synthesized by the lens epithelial cells
   C only superficial cortical lens fibres possess nuclei
   D the basal lens epithelial membrane is rich in Na^+K^+ ATPase pumps
   E the lens interior has an osmolality of 300 mOsm

72 Which of the following statements about the lens are true?

   A Glucose enters the lens by insulin-independent facilitated diffusion.
   B Aerobic glycolysis is responsible for up to 40% of lens energy production.
   C Amino acids are transported into the lens from the aqueous by secondary active co-transport.
   D Sorbitol is produced in the lens during hyperglycaemia.
   E Calcium levels in the lens are 50 times lower than in the aqueous.

73 Regarding crystallins,

   A gamma crystallins are found mainly in the fetal nucleus
   B alpha crystallins are the only crystallins found in the lens epithelium
   C alpha crystallin is found predominantly in the nucleus
   D beta crystallin is the most abundant crystallin
   E gamma crystallin has the highest molecular mass

74 Which of the following statements about the cause of and associations with cataract formation are true?

   A Hypocalcaemia causes cortical cataracts.
   B Reductions of methionine and cysteine levels are found in cataracts.
   C PUVA therapy causes cataract formation.
   D Systemic corticosteroid causes posterior subcapsular cataract.
   E Chlorpromazine causes cataract.

75 How many of the following statements about the lens are correct?

  A The lens has no sensory innervation.
  B The human lens increases in thickness at a rate of about 0.02 mm per year.
  C The anterior radius of curvature is 10 mm.
  D During accommodation, the posterior surface of the lens remains still and the anterior surface of the lens moves forwards toward the cornea.
  E The anterior lens capsule is three times thicker than the posterior capsule.

Vitreous

76 Which of the following statements about the vitreous are true?

  A The vitreous transports low molecular weight substances by diffusion and high molecular weight substances by bulk flow.
  B Collagen provides the major resistance to flow of water in the vitreous.
  C Hyaluronic acid possesses a cationic charge.
  D Zonule fibres like the vitreous collagen fibrils resist collagenase.
  E Age-related liquefaction of the vitreous begins in the central vitreous.

77 The vitreous

  A contains hyaluronic acid produced by hyalocytes
  B is absent of fibroblasts, except in response to trauma
  C shortens the partial thromboplastin time and aggregates platelets
  D provides nutrients for the retina
  E actively replaces 50% of water every 10–15 min

78 How many of the following are true?

  A In the vitreous, collagen density is greatest in the posterior cortex.
  B Cloquet's canal is devoid of collagen fibrils.
  C The vitreous is susceptible to osmotic dehydration through mannitol therapy.
  D The vitreous cortex is thin over the optic disc and absent over the macula.
  E Hyalocytes are found in a single layer anterior to the inner limiting membrane of the retina.

79 The vitreous

  A does not transmit UV light below 400 nm
  B plays a role in the blood–ocular barrier

C has osmolality usually less than that of serum

D potassium levels can be used in forensic medicine in determining the time elapsed since death

E to plasma ratio of ascorbic acid is 2:1

80 The vitreous

A occupies up to 60% of the globe

B has a refractive index similar to that of the aqueous

C is composed mainly of type I collagen

D in the human has no hyaluronic acid before birth

E contains hyaluronic acid concentrated mainly in the cortex

The retina

81 Which of the following statements about the retina are true?

A The central retinal artery only receives sympathetic innervation beyond the lamina cribrosa.

B The central retinal artery beyond the lamina cribrosa displays α-adrenergic receptors.

C Sympathetic innervation increases ocular blood flow.

D The choroidal vessels receive parasympathetic innervation.

E Both retinal and choroidal vessels vasodilate during hypoxia or hypercapnia.

82 In the retina,

A Müller cells are a form of oligodendrocyte

B shedding of rod discs occurs predominantly in the morning

C the foveola is deficient in blue cones

D the external limiting membrane is formed by the zonula occludens of the retinal pigment epithelium

E the inner segment of the photoreceptors receive their blood supply from the central retinal artery

83 With regard to the retina,

A Müller cells are confined by the internal and external limiting membranes

B the inner and outer segments of a photoreceptor are connected by a ciliary stalk consisting of ten pairs of microtubules

C visual pigments are insoluble membrane proteins found on photoreceptor discs

D the 11-*cis*-retinaldehyde in rhodopsin lies parallel to the disc membrane

E the Müller cell is responsible for the b-wave in the electroretinogram

84 How many of the following statements about the retina are correct?

A The Gs protein 'transducin' in the photoreceptors remains inactive due to the presence of the α subunit.

B The retinal pigment epithelium stores photopigment.

C The apicolateral surfaces of the retinal pigment epithelium contains zonula adherens and zonula occludens.

D 11-*cis*-Retinol is oxidized to 11-*cis*-retinaldehyde by 11-*cis*-retinol dehydrogenase in the retinal pigment epithelium.

E All-*trans*-retinaldehyde combines with the apoprotein opsin to form rhodopsin.

85 With regard to the retina,

A cGMP levels in the photoreceptors are low in the dark and rise in response to light

B light exposure results in inhibition of phosphodiesterase

C a 'triad' refers to a penetration of two central dendrites from a bipolar cell and a process from a horizontal cell into a cone pedicle

D the retinal pigment epithelium is a bilayer of cells arranged in a mainly hexagonal array

E photoreceptor tips are attached to retinal pigment epithelium processes by junctional complexes

86 In the retina,

A rhodopsin has a half-life of 10 days

B the 'dark current' refers to the inflow of sodium ions from the extracellular space entering the inner segment of the photoreceptor

C photoreceptors are ON cells

D less than one-fifth of glucose oxidation is via the hexose monophosphate shunt pathway

E the blood flow per unit mass to the retina is three times higher than to the kidney

87 Which of the following are true?

A β-Carotene and retinyl esters are converted to retinol or vitamin A alcohol by the retinal pigment epithelium.

B The only visual pigment reaction requiring light is the conversion of rhodopsin to bathorhodopsin.

C The outer segment of the retina is vulnerable to hypoxia in the dark.

D ATP synthesis is found on the inner membrane on the mitochondria.

E Sixty per cent of glucose metabolism in the retina is by anaerobic glycolysis.

88 Regarding the retina, which of the following are correct?

A Photoreceptors store glycogen.

B Glucose uptake in the retina is insulin independent.

C ON bipolar and OFF bipolar cells both release glutamate and directly excite ganglion cells.

D Pyruvate production in the retina is always greater than pyruvate metabolism.

E Light adaptation is delayed at high altitude.

Electrophysiological investigations

89 Which of the following statements about electroretinography are true?

A The electroretinogram (ERG) is normal if disease is confined to the macula.

B The electro-oculogram (EOG) is abnormal in retinitis pigmentosa.

C The pattern ERG P50 wave is abnormal in disease confined to the macula.

D Visual evoked potential (VEP) may be used to predict location of compressive lesions of the optic nerve.

E The early receptor potential of the ERG only occurs in dim light.

90 With regard to electroretinography and electro-oculography,

A the a-wave of the ERG is absent/abnormal in glaucoma

B 30 Hz flicker ERG produces a pure cone response

C a normal Arden index is less than 180%

D the Arden index refers to the ratio of the light peak and the dark peak of the EOG

E the c-wave of the ERG is produced by the retinal pigment epithelium

91 How many of the following are true?

A ERG is performed using electrodes placed over the visual cortex.

B The pattern ERG is commonly used to confirm central retinal artery occlusion.

C The flash VEP is unaffected by refractive errors.

D The b-wave of the ERG increases in amplitude in dark adaptation.

E Barbiturates reduce the amplitude of the ERG response.

The extraocular muscles

92 Which of the following statements about the extraocular muscles are true?

   A The outer orbital layer of muscle fibres consist mainly of motor end-plates scattered along the whole length of the muscle.
   B Calcium influx for excitation contraction coupling of the global fibres is from the surface membrane and not the sarcoplasmic reticulum.
   C The extraocular muscles display a depolarizing block on exposure to succinyl-choline (suxamethonium) that is enhanced by further exposure to a cholinesterase.
   D Sherrington's law describes the movement of yoke muscles.
   E Concentration of mitochondria is greater in the orbital layer than the global layer of the rectus muscle.

93 With regard to the extraocular muscles,

   A they contain a high number of muscle spindles
   B tertiary positions of gaze involve rotation about the Y-axis
   C torsion by obliques involves rotation about the Y-axis
   D in the isolated agonist model, the primary action of superior oblique is of depression and abduction
   E inferior oblique causes intorsion

PHYSIOLOGY
Answers

General physiology

Cardiovascular

1 **A** = True   **B** = False   **C** = False   **D** = True   **E** = True   **F** = True   **G** = False

Cardiac output is the volume expelled by the left ventricle per unit time. It is heart rate $\times$ stroke volume and can be determined using Fick's principle:

$$\text{Cardiac output} = \text{oxygen consumption } (V_{O_2}) \text{ divided by}$$
$$\text{arteriovenous } O_2 \text{ concentration difference } (avD_{O_2})$$

Cardiac output is usually calculated by thermodilution. Haemoglobin concentration is not required in order to calculate cardiac output.

As a unit volume of blood passes successively through the aorta, large arteries, major branches, arterioles and capillaries, velocity decreases progressively as the total cross-sectional area increases. The velocity of flow is inversely proportionally to the total cross-sectional area of the vessels. The flow is usually laminar (streamline) in large vessels, with greatest velocity being in the centre of the flow. At a critical velocity flow changes from the silent streamline to the noisy turbulent flow (i.e. bruits, Korotkoff sounds).

In anaemia, turbulence is seen due to reduced viscosity (haematocrit) and so increased velocity of flow. The Hagen–Poiseuille Law explains that resistance to flow is proportional to the length of a tube (L) and the viscosity of the fluid (n), and inversely proportional to the fourth power of the radius.

Blood flow in systole may be as high as 0.7 m/s in the aorta but compliance of the aortic vessel wall causes stretch followed by rebound. Blood flows in diastole with a smooth type of flow and an overall mean velocity of 0.2 m/s.

Coronary blood flow at rest is 250 ml/min (5% of cardiac output) and during exercise can rise up to 750 ml/min, remaining approximately 5% of cardiac output. Increased coronary oxygen consumption is further facilitated by a greater avD_{O_2}.

2 **A** = False   **B** = False   **C** = False   **D** = False   **E** = True   **F** = True

Blood flow depends on vessel diameter which is influenced and regulated by local, neural and hormonal control.

Myogenic autoregulation describes vasoconstriction secondary to a rise in blood pressure causing vessels to stretch. Renal and cerebral blood flow are controlled by autoregulation and are influenced by this myogenic effect. Skin and pulmonary vessels are not regulated by myogenic autoregulation.

Hypoxic autoregulation describes vasodilation in response to low levels of oxygen, thereby allowing increased blood flow and oxygen supply. Most vessels vasodilate in the presence of hypoxia, however pulmonary vessels undergo *hypoxic vasoconstriction* which facilitates blood to lung areas of greater ventilation in oxygenation. Note that vasoconstriction of greater than 50% of pulmonary vasculature results in pulmonary hypertension.

Increased local levels of metabolites such as CO_2 (especially skin and brain) and H^+ (decreased pH), ADP, AMP, adenosine (cardiac muscle not skeletal) and K^+ (especially skeletal) cause vasodilation (*reactive hyperaemia*) to facilitate faster removal. A rise in local temperature also causes a vasodilation as does the release of EDRF (endothelium-derived relaxing factor) which is now known to be nitric oxide.

There is *neural control* of both vasoconstriction and vasodilation. The arterioles in the skeletal muscles circulation are mainly under control of β_2-adrenergic receptors; however, the increased blood flow observed in exercise is mainly due to vasodilation secondary to the accumulation of tissue metabolites.

3 **A** = False   **B** = False   **C** = True   **D** = True   **E** = False   **F** = True

Between 0.3 and 0.5% of plasma flow is filtered by capillaries into the interstitial space. This is calculated by cardiac output being 5 L/min, therefore 7200 L a day. Haematocrit is 0.45, therefore plasma flow is 3960 L a day. It is known that approximately 20–24 L of fluid each day enters the interstitial space through capillaries outside the kidneys, thus a calculation of 0.3–0.5% can be made. Ninety per cent of this ultrafiltrate is resorbed through the capillaries back into the circulation. Ten per cent returns via lymph.

At heart level, precapillary hydrostatic pressure is 30 mmHg, falling to 14 mmHg at the venous end. The oncotic pressure difference is about 20 mmHg. This decreases with increasing capillary permeability. Starling's hypothesis explains that this difference along with available area of exchange determines the extent of transcapillary filtration and resorption. In most organs the capillary wall is almost completely impermeable to protein. Permeability is greater, however, in the liver and also the intestines.

As blood passes through capillaries, fluid filters out into the interstitial space. Haematocrit therefore increases as blood undergoes haemoconcentration. CO_2 formed by metabolism dissolves readily in the interstitial space and diffuses into the red blood cells. It is converted to HCO_3^- and H^+ quickly by carbonic anhydrase. H^+ is buffered in the cell and HCO_3^- diffuses passively into the plasma in exchange for Cl^- diffusing into the red cells. The greater concentration of Cl^- in venous red cells than in arterial red cells results in a fluid shift into the red cell, thereby increasing mean cell volume.

The Bohr effect describes how a fall in pH reduces the affinity of haemoglobin for oxygen. For a given Po_2, a reduction in percentage saturation of haemoglobin and oxygen-carrying capacity of blood is seen. The oxygen–haemoglobin dissociation curve shifts to the right.

4 **A** = False **B** = False **C** = False **D** = False **E** = False

Baroreceptors are stretch receptors. They are found in blood vessel walls over the aortic arch and carotid sinus. They are also found in the walls of left ventricle, left and right atria, the superior vena cava and the inferior vena cava as well as the pulmonary veins. They discharge with stretch and inhibit sympathetic vasoconstrictor activity and stimulate vagal cardiac activity. Blood pressure decreases by vasodilation, bradycardia and a fall in cardiac output. Venodilation also occurs.

5 **A** = False **B** = False **C** = False **D** = True **E** = False

Vasodilation during erection in genital organs is due to parasympathetic stimulation by postganglionic cholinergic fibres. Adrenaline vasodilates in low concentrations by its effect on β_2 receptors in skeletal muscle and the liver. In high concentrations it is a vasoconstrictor by acting on α receptors.

ADH (vasopressin) is a potent vasoconstrictor *in vitro*.

Pain via afferent impulses to the reticular formation acts on the vasomotor centre causing raised blood pressure.

Inspiration causes increased venous return to the right side of the heart and reduced venous return to the left side of the heart. This in turn briefly reduces left ventricular output. Also, via vagal afferent signals there is a brief inhibition of the vasomotor centre causing vasodilation and a transient fall in blood pressure. This fall in blood pressure is detected by baroreceptors that trigger activation of the vaso- motor centre and reduce activation of the vagal cardioinhibitory centre in compensa- tion. The process of inspiration and expiration thus causes a physiological sinus arrythmia.

6 **A** = False **B** = False **C** = True **D** = False **E** = False

Pulse pressure is the difference in systolic and diastolic pressure. It is a function of arterial compliance and stroke volume. It rises with increased vessel rigidity (decreased compliance) and increased stroke volume. Mean pressure is proportional to total peripheral resistance. It is the geometric mean of systolic and diastolic pressure, or roughly equates to the diastolic plus one-third of the difference between systolic and diastolic pressure.

Pulmonary artery pressure is approximately 25 mmHg (13.3 kPa) systolic and 10 mmHg (1.3 kPa) diastolic. Mean pressure is therefore approximately 15 mmHg.

Conditions causing chronic hypoxia such as living at high altitudes and chronic obstructive airways disease, cause pulmonary hypoxic vasoconstriction in order to compensate for a ventilation: perfusion mismatch. Vasoconstriction of greater than 50% of the pulmonary vasculature raises resistance enough to cause pulmonary hypertension.

Blood pressure may be measured directly by placing sensory devices directly into the arterial blood stream, and indirectly by using an inflatable cuff.

7 **A** = False   **B** = False   **C** = False   **D** = False   **E** = False

The phases of the cardiac cycle are: (1) systolic contraction phase; (2) systolic ejection phase; (3) relaxation phase of diastole; (4) diastolic filling phase.

End-diastolic ventricular volume is approximately 125 ml, which can double in exercise. The ventricular filling at rest is mainly passive. Atrial contraction contributes to the final 20%, but at higher heart rates, because diastole is shorter, it contributes more.

Systole begins with a contraction phase, initially with isovolumetric contraction: ventricular pressure rises with fixed volume. Once ventricular pressure is greater than aortic pressure, the next phase of ejection proceeds by opening of the semilunar valves.

Coronary blood flow to the left ventricle occurs only in diastole because the left ventricular walls squeeze the vessels during contraction. Pressure in the right ventricle only reaches up to 25 mmHg. For this reason, coronary blood flow to the right ventricle mainly occurs in diastole but also occurs at a reduced rate in systole.

The jugular venous pulse is made of five main waves: a, c, x, v, y. The positive a-wave represents atrial contraction. This is followed by a second positive c-wave, representing closure of the tricuspid valve. The negative x-wave represents a fall in venous pressure as contraction in the ventricle pulls the valves and results in depression of their level. This creates a 'suction effect' in the great veins. Next is the positive v-wave representing the opening of the tricuspid valve forced by a rise in the atrial pressure (filling). The final negative y-wave represents passive filling of blood from the atrium to the ventricle.

8 **A** = True   **B** = True   **C** = True   **D** = False   **E** = False

The Frank–Starling Law describes how the 'energy of muscle contraction is related to the initial length of the cardiac muscle fibre'. The initial length is proportional to end-diastolic volume and if plotted against stroke volume gives the Frank–Starling curve. Lying supine rather than standing increases venous return to the heart as does venous contraction. Ventricular filling occurs in diastole and is reduced in tachycardia. Cardiac tamponade causes reduced ventricular volume.

9 **A** = False   **B** = False   **C** = False   **D** = True   **E** = True   **F** = True

Foetal placental blood has an oxygen saturation of 80%. Oxygenated blood is carried from the placenta in the umbilical vein through the ductus venosus, bypassing the liver, to the inferior vena cava and the heart.

The ductus arteriosus carries venous blood largely from the superior vena cava entering the right ventricle and pulmonary artery through to the aorta. At birth the direction of flow reverses. It closes a few days after birth.

The umbilical artery carries deoxygenated blood from the foetus to the placenta.

At birth, sudden loss of the placenta results in an increased CO_2 and other waste products. The rise in P_{CO_2} stimulates ventilation via chemoreceptors.

Respiratory

10 **A** = True   **B** = False   **C** = False   **D** = False   **E** = True   **F** = True

Dry air at sea level has an atmospheric pressure of 760 mmHg (101.3 kPa), P_{N_2} = 601 mmHg (80.1 kPa), P_{O_2} = 159 mmHg (21.2 kPa) and P_{CO_2} = 0.23 mmHg (0.03 kPa).

Before reaching the alveoli, expired area is humidified by the trachea and P_{H_2O} is at the constant value of 47 mmHg (6.37 kPa). This results in alveolar P_{N_2} = 574 mmHg (76.5 kPa), P_{O_2} = 100 mmHg (13.3 kPa), P_{CO_2} = 39 mmHg (5.2 kPa) and P_{H_2O} = 47 mmHg (6.27 kPa).

Physiological arteriovenous shunting due to ventilation: perfusion mismatching and bronchial veins carrying deoxygenated blood into the oxygenated pulmonary vein causes arterial blood gases different to those of alveoli.

In the aorta P_{O_2} = 95 mmHg (12.66 kPa) and P_{CO_2} = 41 mmHg (5.47 kPa).

Mixed venous blood P_{O_2} = 40 mmHg (5.33 kPa), P_{CO_2} = 45 mmHg (6.0 kPa).

Expired air P_{O_2} = 115 mmHg (15.33 kPa), P_{CO_2} = 33 mmHg (4.4 kPa), P_{H_2O} = 47 mmHg (6.27 kPa), P_{N_2} = 565 mmHg (76.5 kPa). Note that the fractional concentrations of expired air are O_2 = 0.14–0.15%, CO_2 = 0.45%, H_2O = 0.06% and N_2 = 0.75%.

11 **A** = False   **B** = False   **C** = False   **D** = True   **E** = False   **F** = True   **G** = False
   H = True

Lung surfactant decreases alveolar surface tension.

Dead space refers to the total volume of air channels transmitting inspired air to the alveoli and not taking part in gas exchange (i.e. mouth, nose, pharynx, trachea and bronchi). Physiological dead space refers to anatomical dead space plus any areas of reduced gas exchange either by reducing perfusion to alveoli or by impairing diffusion across alveolar membranes, thereby creating further dead space. Physiological dead space is at least equal to anatomical dead space, but may well be greater. Pulmonary embolus impairs lung perfusion, creating a ventilation: perfusion mismatch and increases physiological dead space.

Tidal volume (V_T) equals volume reaching alveoli (V_A) plus air shifted in dead space (V_D). Dead space is approximately 150 ml. It may be calculated using the Bohr equation.

Tidal volume equals 500 ml, therefore the volume reaching alveoli is approximately 350 ml.

If *f* is the frequency of breathing, then:

$$V_T.f = V_A.f + V_D.f$$

In rapid shallow breathing V_T is reduced as frequency increases. Minute ventilation ($V_T.f$) increases slightly; however, as dead space (V_D) remains constant the result is that dead space ventilation ($V_D.f$) is increased markedly and alveolar ventilation ($V_A f$) and gas exchange are reduced.

12 **A** = True   **B** = False   **C** = True   **D** = False   **E** = False   **F** = True

The lungs have a tendency to contract, causing intrapleural pressure to be negative. Intrapleural pressure becomes positive mainly in forced expiration.

Pulmonary compliance is changed in volume per unit of change in transpulmonary pressure.

Compliance is the reciprocal of elastance. It is increased in emphysema because of loss of elasticity and an enlargement of respiratory bronchioles and alveoli, and break-down of alveolar walls.

Alveoli are lined with two types of epithelial cells: type I cells are the primary lining of the alveoli and are flat with lots of cytoplasm; type II cells (or granular pneumocytes) are thicker, contain inclusion bodies, and produce surfactant.

13 **A** = False   **B** = False   **C** = False   **D** = True   **E** = True

Vital capacity (V_C) is the volume expired from maximum inspiration to maximum expiration. V_C = 4.5 L, however varies from 2.5 to 7 L according to height, age, sex and physical training.

Tidal volume (V_T) is the volume inspired during quiet respiration. V_T = 0.5 L.

Inspiratory reserve volume (IRV) is the volume of gas inspired by expiration at rest to full inspiration. IRV = 3 L.

Expiratory reserve volume (ERV) is the volume expired from expiration at rest to full expiration. ERV = 1.5 L.

Residual volume (RV) is the volume of gas remaining in the lungs after full expiration. RV = 1.5 L.

Functional residual capacity (FRC) is the volume of gas remaining in lungs after expiration at rest. FRC = 3 L.

Total lung capacity (TLC) is the vital capacity plus residual volume. V_C + RV = TLC = 6 L. This varies with age, sex, size and physical training.

V_C, V_T, IRV and ERV may be measured using spirometry. RV and FRC must be measured indirectly using helium or nitrogen dilution, or whole-body plethysmography (to also include encapsulated air spaces such as cysts etc.). See Figure 1.

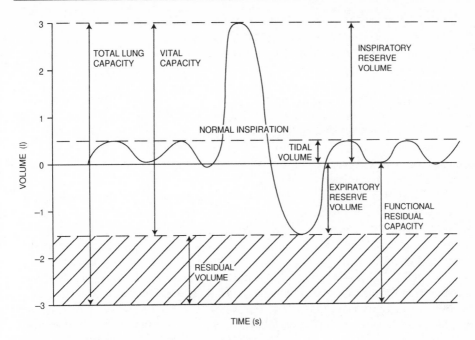

Figure 1 Parameters used to calculate respiratory volumes

14 A = False **B** = True **C** = True **D** = True **E** = False

Lung surfactant is made up of dipalmitoylphosphatidylcholine, other phospholipids, lipids and proteins. It lowers surface tension in the walls of alveoli, increasing compliance and preventing collapse. It is reduced in hyaline membrane disease and heavy smoking.

The Laplace relationship defines surface tension in the wall of a sphere as being proportional to transmural pressure times radius. For a given fluid lining the sphere the surface tension is constant and so pressure across the wall reduces as radius increases.

15 A = False **B** = False **C** = True **D** = True **E** = False

Alveolar ventilation is greater in the base of the lung compared to the apex when upright. This is because the apex is already expanded due to stretch as a result of the weight of the lung before inspiration begins. The base of the lung has a greater volume of expansion during inspiration. When erect, the pulmonary blood flow (per unit volume) increases from apex to base. When supine, this difference disappears.

Due to ventilation increasing less steeply than pulmonary blood flow from apex to base, the ventilation: perfusion ratio is greater in the apex (3.3) than the base (0.63) of the lung when erect.

Transection of the spinal cord above the level of C3 is fatal as both phrenic nerves are lost as well as the innervation to the intercostal muscles.

Physiological dead space causes a high ventilation:perfusion ratio.

16 **A** = True   **B** = False   **C** = False   **D** = False   **E** = False

CO_2 is approximately 20 times more soluble than O_2 in blood. Deoxygenated haemoglobin binds CO_2 more readily than does oxyhaemoglobin. This allows CO_2 to be carried away from tissue in venous blood and results in release of CO_2 in the pulmonary capillaries where haemoglobin is then oxygenated.

CO_2 diffuses easily across the blood–brain barrier. H^+ and HCO_3^-, however, do not diffuse easily across the blood–brain barrier.

Carotid body chemoreceptors respond primarily to changes in P_{O_2}.

The majority of CO_2 in blood is distributed as HCO_3^-. CO_2 diffusing into a red blood cell is converted quickly into HCO_3^- by the enzyme carbonic anhydrase. Seventy per cent of this HCO_3^- leaves the red blood cell in exchange for Cl^- entering. In arterial blood, 3% of CO_2 is dissolved in plasma and 2% is dissolved in the red blood cell; 0.5% is bound to plasma proteins and 5% is bound to haemoglobin in the red blood cell; 60% is distributed as HCO_3^- dissolved in plasma and 30% as HCO_3^- in the red blood cell.

In venous blood the distribution remains relatively similar with CO_2 bound to haemoglobin increasing to up to 6%. The rise in the CO_2 level is reflected in the HCO_3^- concentration in venous blood being higher.

17 **A** = False   **B** = False   **C** = False   **D** = True   **E** = True

Mixed venous blood is 75% saturated with O_2.

Cyanosis is due to the dark colour of deoxygenated haemoglobin which gives skin a bluish-grey discoloration. It occurs when the concentration of deoxygenated haemoglobin in blood is greater than 5 g/100 ml and is due to the absolute concentration. It occurs in polycythaemia in the absence of tissue hypoxia.

Hypoxia stimulates peripheral (carotid) chemoreceptors. A rise in P_{CO_2} stimulates central chemoreceptors and also sensitizes the peripheral chemoreceptors to changes in P_{O_2}.

The oxygen dissociation curve is a sigmoid curve with the x-axis being P_{O_2} and the y-axis being either O_2 saturation or concentration of oxygenated haemoglobin. It may be displaced to the left or right as well as 'stretched' vertically when describing oxyhaemoglobin concentration (O_2 capacity) with haemoglobin fully saturated.

The curve is shifted to the left (increased O_2 affinity) by a rise in pH (decreased $[H^+]$ – the Bohr effect), a fall in temperature and a fall in the levels of 2,3-diphosphoglycerate (2,3-DPG) in the red blood cells. The curve is shifted to the right with the opposite conditions.

2,3-DPG is the product of anaerobic glycolysis and is found in the red blood cells. It is anionic and binds avidly to deoxyhaemoglobin. Increased levels are seen during exercise, altitude and anaemia that may cause hypoxia.

A rise in 2,3-DPG is seen to facilitate oxygen release from haemoglobin to the tissues. Storing blood results in reduced glycolysis and reduced 2,3–DPG production. This results in a shift to the left of the oxygen dissociation curve and reduced oxygen release from haemoglobin.

Renal

18 **A** = True   **B** = False   **C** = False   **D** = True   **E** = False

The kidneys have three main roles: (1) an excretory role, (2) a homeostatic role, and (3) an endocrine role, whereby they produce hormones including renin, erythropoietin and 1α-hydroxylase.

1α-Hydroxylase is a crucial enzyme in the final step in production of 1,25-dihydroxycholecalciferol (calcitriol) from 25-hydroxycholecalciferol. Calcitriol plays an important role in calcium and skeletal mineralization.

The cells of the proximal convoluted tubule possess a rich brush border and numerous mitochondria beside the basolateral membrane. The distal convoluted tubules are poor in mitochondria and do not possess a brush border. The macula densa exists early on at the distal convoluted tubule.

19 **A** = True   **B** = False   **C** = False   **D** = True   **E** = False   **F** = False

Renal blood flow at rest is 25% of cardiac output (1.2 L/min). The renal artery divides into interlobar arteries, then into arcuate arteries, then into interlobular arteries in the cortex of the kidney, finally dividing into afferent arterioles. Autoregulation of renal blood flow occurs mainly at the level of the afferent arteriole. The interlobular arteries play a role in controlling renal blood flow and are highly sensitive to local catecholamines. The efferent arterioles are constricted by angiotensin II and improve perfusion when pressure is low.

Autoregulation maintains constant renal blood flow with mean arterial blood pressure between 80 and 200 mmHg. Mean arterial blood pressure may be roughly calculated as diastolic plus one-third of the difference between systolic and diastolic.

The kidneys filter plasma rather than blood. Plasma volume = blood volume × (1 − haematocrit). Renal plasma flow can be measured using Fick's principle by measuring the amount of a given substance removed per unit time divided by the arteriovenous difference in concentration.

Para-aminohippuric acid is useful in calculating renal blood flow as it is filtered by the glomerulus and further secreted into the proximal convoluted tubule. It is also reliable because at low-dose infusions 90% is cleared in each single renal circulation.

20 **A** = True   **B** = False   **C** = False   **D** = False   **E** = True   **F** = False   **G** = True

The glomerular filtration rate in a normal adult is approximately 125 ml/min (both kidneys). It is proportional to body surface area. As renal plasma flow is approximately 700 ml/min, GFR is calculated as being 20% of renal plasma flow. GFR of 125 ml/min is equivalent to 180 L/day and 99% of this is reabsorbed in the tubules to produce approximately 1 L of urine per day. Twenty per cent of GFR would be 36 L of urine a day, which is clearly not seen.

Diabetes insipidus is a result of the absence or ineffective action of ADH acting on the distal convoluting tubule and collecting ducts.

Blood urea concentration is a poor test of glomerular function, because although a normal concentration relies on renal excretion, it also depends on dietary protein intake.

Inulin clearance is useful in measuring the GFR because it is freely filtered by the glomerulus and is not bound to plasma protein. It is not reabsorbed or secreted by tubule cells and is not stored or metabolized. It is non-toxic, does not actually effect the glomerular filtration rate and is relatively easy to measure in both plasma and urine.

21 **A** = True   **B** = True   **C** = True   **D** = False   **E** = False

D-Glucose is reabsorbed only in the proximal convoluted tubule mainly in the early part. The mechanism is by secondary active co-transport whereby it is coupled with Na^+ transport into the cell. Na^+ transport into the cell is along a concentration gradient created by the Na^+K^+ ATPase pump situated on the basolateral membrane of the tubular epithelium.

Uric acid is predominantly reabsorbed at the proximal convoluted tubule; however, small quantities of uric acid, endogenous substances such as glucororides, and exogenous substances such as PAH and penicillin and other drugs are actively secreted into the proximal convoluted tubule.

Potassium and H^+ ions are actively secreted in both proximal and distal convoluted tubules and the collecting ducts. Creatinine is actively secreted in small amounts by the proximal convoluted tubules and increases total creatinine in urine by up to 20%.

The tubular epithelium is impermeable to urea except for the proximal convoluted tubule and the medullary portion of the collecting ducts, where urea passively moves out along an osmotic gradient.

Although natural penicillins are metabolized to a small extent to the inactive penicilloic acid by hydrolysis of the β-lactam ring in either the gastrointestinal tract or the liver, they are mainly and rapidly excreted in urine by tubular secretion.

Two-thirds of a single intramuscular or intravenous dose of penicillin G is excreted mainly unchanged within 6 h. Over 90% of this is by active tubular secretion and 10% by glomerular filtration.

Approximately half of a single oral dose of penicillin V is excreted in urine within 8 h and approximately 30% is excreted in faeces.

22 A = False **B** = True **C** = True **D** = False **E** = True

Sodium reabsorption does not occur on the descending loop of Henle. Seventy per cent of sodium is reabsorbed in the proximal convoluted tubule actively due to the basolateral Na^+K^+ ATPase pump. Cl^- and H_2O follow by secondary active transport and an osmotic gradient respectively, resulting in isotonic resorption.

In the thick ascending loop, a further 20% is reabsorbed by the basolateral Na^+K^+ ATPase pump, creating a sodium gradient for sodium to enter from the luminal side. The sodium enters the thick ascending loop tubule cells via a carrier channel, the Na^+-K^+ and $2Cl^-$ channel by a process of secondary active co-transport. Loop diuretics inhibit this channel and in doing so prevent a concentration gradient being created in the renal medulla.

Carbonic anhydrase inhibitors are useful diuretic agents. They inhibit the reversible $HCO_3^- + H^+ \rightleftharpoons CO_2 + H_2O$.

Filtered HCO_3^- is normally converted to CO_2 and H_2O by luminal brush border carbonic anhydrase at the proximal convoluted tubule. The CO_2 and H_2O passively enter the tubule cells and carbonic anhydrase in the tubular cells produces HCO_3^- and H^+ again. H^+ may be excreted coupled to sodium reabsorption and HCO_3^- is reabsorbed into the circulation by secondary active transport. Inhibition of carbonic anhydrase essentially inhibits this process. This reduces the sodium reabsorption that is coupled with H^+ excretion, but more importantly inhibits HCO_3^- reabsorption. Reduced H^+ excretion results in increased potassium excretion as potassium and H^+ compete with each other.

Aldosterone, by acting on DNA and modifying protein synthesis at the distal convoluted tubule, collecting ducts and to a small degree the bladder, increases sodium reabsorption within 30 min.

23 A = True **B** = True **C** = True **D** = False **E** = True

The weight of a 70 kg man is made up of 60% water (42 L) and 40% proteins, minerals and fat. Of the body water content, two-thirds (40% total weight or 28 L) is intracellular and one-third (20% weight or 14 L) is extracellular. Of the extracellular fluid, three-quarters (15% weight or approximately 10.5 L) is in the interstitial space, whereas one-quarter (5% weight or approximately 3.5 L) makes up plasma volume.

Intracellular and extracellular fluid osmolality is 290 mOsm/kg H_2O. Extracellular fluid osmolality is tightly controlled by hypothalamic osmoreceptors which stimulate hypothalamic production and posterior pituitary release of ADH, with effects on the target organ, the kidney.

A rise of 3 mOsm/kg H_2O (1%) is all that is needed to increase ADH release. Pain also increases ADH release. ADH release is inhibited by intake of hypotonic fluid such as water, causing a fall in osmolality. Reduced sodium intake resulting in reduced osmolality may briefly reduce ADH release. Alcohol inhibits ADH release.

24 **A** = True   **B** = True   **C** = False   **D** = True   **E** = False

Renin is an enzyme produced and stored as pro-renin by the juxtaglomerular cells of the kidney (but also produced in the brain, heart and adrenal gland). It is released as renin and cleaves angiotensinogen (from the liver) to produce angiotensin I (a decapeptide). Angiotensin I is converted to the active angiotensin II by converting enzymes found in the lungs, kidneys and elsewhere. Angiotensin II acts to elevate arterial blood pressure both by rapid vasoconstriction at the level of the arterioles and by reducing salt and water excretion by the kidneys.

Angiotensin II acts on the kidneys both directly and indirectly. Directly, its mechanism is thought to be vasoconstriction of renal vasculature and a weak effect on tubules increasing reabsorption of sodium and water. Indirectly, angiotensin II stimulates increased aldosterone production at the zona glomerulosa of the adrenal cortex.

Aldosterone acts mainly to increase sodium and water reabsorption at the distal convoluted tubules and collecting ducts of the kidney. This causes a rise in extracellular volume and helps to maintain raised arterial blood pressure.

Hypoaldosteronism results in hyponatraemia and hyperkalaemia; however, hyperaldosteronism results in a normal sodium concentration as a result of the consequent water reabsorption, and instead, hypokalaemia as a result of increased potassium excretion.

Endocrinology

25 **A** = True   **B** = True   **C** = True   **D** = True   **E** = True

Iodine deficiency (and paradoxically excess as well) inhibits thyroid function, leading to primary hypothyroidism where TSH secretion increases due to the lack of negative feedback. Thyroxine increases oxygen uptake and consumption in most cells of the body. Although not essential to life, it is necessary for normal growth and development and regulates lipid and carbohydrate metabolism.

Hypercholesterolaemia is seen in hypothyroidism. This is thought to be because thyroxine increases low density lipoprotein (LDL) receptor formation in the liver, thus facilitating removal of circulating cholesterol.

Iodide is taken up by TSH-independently in the salivary glands, gastric mucosa, ciliary body of the eye, choroid plexus, placenta and mammary glands.

The half-life of thyroxine is approximately 6–7 days.

26 **A** = True   **B** = False   **C** = True   **D** = True   **E** = True   **F** = False

Ninety-nine per cent of circulating T4 is bound either to plasma or tissue proteins. These plasma proteins include:

1 thyroxine-binding globulin (TBG), which although present in small concentrations binds 67% of T4;

2 thyroxine-binding pre-albumin (TBPA), which binds 15% of T4;

3 albumin, which binds 13% of T4.

Thyroid hormones enter cells without binding to receptors or channels. They bind to nuclear membrane receptors and the resulting thyroid receptor complex then binds to DNA altering gene expression. The change in mRNA produced causes production of enzymes that are able to alter cell function. T3 and T4 are able to cross the blood–brain barrier and are found in grey matter. CSF protein levels are raised in hypothyroidism and lowered in hyperthyroidism.

The half-life of TSH is 1 h. TSH is secreted in a pulsatile form. It begins to increase from 21.00 hours and peaks at approximately midnight, declining during the day.

Regulation of thyroid secretion is by a negative feedback mechanism. TRH from the hypothalamus directly stimulates TSH release from the anterior pituitary. TSH increases iodide uptake and T3/T4 production by the thyroid gland. Free T3 and T4 in the circulation directly inhibit both TRH production by the hypothalamus and TSH production by the anterior pituitary. T3 is more active than T4, as it binds more readily and acts more rapidly and effectively than T4 on the nuclear receptor. T4 is converted in the periphery to T3 by deiodination.

27 **A** = True **B** = True **C** = True **D** = True **E** = False

Glucagon is a catabolic hormone produced in the A cells in the Islets of Langerhans as pre-proglucagon. It is useful in mobilizing stores of glucose, fatty acids and amino acids. It is made up of a single polypeptide chain and its structure is the same in all mammals. It has a half-life of 5–10 min and is destroyed in the liver.

28 **A** = False **B** = True **C** = False **D** = False **E** = False

Insulin is a 51 amino acid dipeptide with a half-life of 10–30 min. Its actions are generally anabolic, increasing glucose, fatty acid and amino acid stores. It does not increase glucose uptake in the brain, kidney, gastrointestinal mucosa and the red blood cells. Its actions also include a rapid increase in the number of membrane glucose transporter proteins that facilitate glucose uptake into cells. Its immediate effects include increased protein synthesis, glycogenesis and reduced protein breakdown. Its delayed effect is to increase lipogenesis and decrease lipolysis. Insulin inhibits gluconeogenesis in the liver.

29 **A** = False **B** = False **C** = False **D** = False **E** = True

ADH (vasopressin) is a neural hormone from the neurohypophysis. It is produced in the cell bodies of the magnocellular neurones in the supraoptic and paraventricular nuclei of the hypothalamus. ADH is transferred by axoplasmic flow in granules down the axons of these nerves to their nerve endings in the posterior pituitary where they are stored and released in response to an action potential. Its main effects are of water retention by increasing water permeability at the collecting ducts of the kidney. *In vitro* it causes vasoconstriction. It decreases cardiac output when injected *in vivo* by acting on the area postrema.

ADH also acts on the liver to cause glycogenolysis and on the anterior pituitary to increase ACTH release.

ADH release is increased by a fall in extracellular fluid volume, pain and an increase in plasma osmolality of 3 mOsm/kg H_2O.

30 **A** = False   **B** = False   **C** = True   **D** = True   **E** = False

The adrenal medulla is not under regulation of the pituitary. It is supplied by preganglionic sympathetic fibres and is also influenced by the adrenal cortex. Aldosterone is important in the regulation of salt balance and extracellular volume. It is not directly controlled by the pituitary and hypophysectomy does not effect aldosterone release in the same way as cortisol and sex hormones are affected where atrophy of the zona fasciculata and zona reticularis of the adrenal gland is seen.

ACTH is a 39 amino acid peptide hormone derived from the prohormone pro-opiomelanocortin (POMC). It has a half-life of 10 min and is secreted by the anterior pituitary in pulsatile bursts with a mean peak at around 6 am.

Hypertension due to excess growth hormone is caused by increased heart size resulting in increased stroke volume and cardiac output.

LH, FSH, TSH and HCG are two-unit structures made up of an α and a β subunit. ACTH, prolactin and growth hormone have a single-unit chain peptide structure.

31 **A** = True   **B** = True   **C** = True   **D** = False   **E** = False

Hypercalcaemia has many causes. In the presence of reduced serum phosphate, causes can include primary hyperparathyroidism, tertiary hyperparathyroidism or ectopic parathyroid secretion. Hypercalcaemia associated with raised serum phosphate may be due to excess vitamin D (due to over-administration, sarcoidosis or idiopathic), malignancy of bone (including osteolytic bone metastases, secretion of PTH-like peptide, and myeloma), thiazide diuretic therapy (that promotes calcium absorption) or hyperthyroidism.

Effects of hypercalcaemia include cardiovascular (increased digoxin toxicity, sudden arrest, hypertension), gastrointestinal (gastric ulcers, constipation, abdominal pain), neurological (depression, anorexia, nausea and vomiting) and renal (polyuria) effects.

Hypocalcaemia associated with hyperphosphataemia may be due to primary hypoparathyroidism as a result of surgery to the thyroid or parathyroids. It may also be due to chronic renal failure or be seen in shock with hypoalbuminaemia. It may be associated with secondary hyperparathyroidism or be due to acute pancreatitis or reduced intake of vitamin D.

Effects of hypocalcaemia include paresthesia, numbness, cramps, anxiety, convulsions, laryngeal stridor, dystonia and psychosis.

32 A = True   **B** = True   **C** = False   **D** = True   **E** = False

A 70 kg adult contains approximately 1.1 kg of calcium, 99% of which is in the skeletal cortex. Calcitonin is produced by the parafollicular C cells of the thyroid gland and is secreted in response to hypercalcaemia.

Parathyroid hormone increases renal tubular reabsorption of calcium and loss of phosphate. It also increases cortical bone reabsorption and by stimulating 1α-hydroxylase activity in the kidney, it increases hydroxylation of 25-OH vitamin D to 1,25-$(OH)_2$ vitamin D.

Oestrogen is known to inhibit osteoclast acitivity in bone; however, no oestrogen receptors have been found in bone.

33 A = True   **B** = False   **C** = False   **D** = True   **E** = True   **F** = true   **G** = True

Renal effects of glucocorticoids include a mineralocorticoid effect of increased sodium reabsorption at the distal convoluted tubule and collecting duct and an increase in the GFR, causing a conflicting increased sodium load.

Unlike aldosterone, glucocorticoids in circulation are mostly bound to an α-globulin known as transcortin or corticosteroid binding globulin (CBG). Some is also bound to albumin.

Effects of glucocorticoids on the immune system include inhibition of lymphocyte formation and so reduction in B and T lymphocytes, reduction in eosinophils, reduction in protein synthesis, reducing production of arachidonic acid derivatives and membrane stabilization reducing histamine release. Phaeochromocytoma describes an adrenal medullary tumour that usually secretes noradrenaline, but can be found to secrete mainly adrenaline.

The aldosterone receptor, being a steroid hormone receptor, is intracellular.

The adrenal cortex secretes 21-carbon and 19-carbon steroids. Aldosterone (zona glomerulosa) and cortisol (zona fasciculata) are 21-carbon steroids and so both have mineralocorticoid activity. Aldosterone has a hydroxyl group at position 18 and so is known as an 18-hydroxycorticosteroid.

34 A = True   **B** = True   **C** = False   **D** = False   **E** = False

Synthesis of noradrenaline and adrenaline involves the conversion of phenylalanine to tyrosine to DOPA to dopamine and to noradrenaline, and then to adrenaline. The half-life of noradrenaline and adrenaline in plasma circulation is approximately 2 min.

The effects of adrenaline on the circulation are mediated by both α- and β-receptors. These effects include increased myocardial contractility, heart rate and excitability. At low concentrations adrenaline causes vasodilation in skeletal muscle and liver vessels and as a result reduces peripheral vascular resistance. Adrenaline also causes an increased cardiac output and wider pulse pressure by increasing systolic and decreasing diastolic arterial blood pressure (mixed α- and β-receptor activity).

The effect of circulating noradrenaline on the heart is similar, but noradrenaline causes generalized vasoconstriction (α-receptor activity). This results in a rise in mean arterial blood pressure by increasing both systolic and diastolic pressure. Secondary to baroceptor stimulation, a compensatory reduction in the heart rate may be seen.

Circulating adrenaline and noradrenaline are mainly broken down in the liver to met-products, conjugates and VMA (3–metho-4–hydroxymandelic acid). Almost 50% of these breakdown products are excreted in urine as met-products, 35% as VMA and small amounts of free noradrenaline and adrenaline are also seen.

5-HIAA (5-hydroxyindoleacetic acid) is the main urinary metabolyte of 5-HT (serotonin).

Adrenalectomy results in reduced plasma levels of adrenaline but not of noradrenaline, whose levels are extremely low and rarely reach those that cause cardiovascular effect. The effects of noradrenaline are mainly due to local release from postganglionic sympathetic nerve endings.

CNS

35 **A** = False   **B** = False   **C** = True   **D** = True   **E** = True   **F** = True   **G** = False

Absorption of CSF at the arachnoid villi is due to hydrostatic pressure and bulk flow. CSF protein content is approximately 20–40 mg/100 ml, resulting in a CSF/plasma ratio of approximately 0.3%. The P_{CO_2} of CSF is approximately 50 mmHg, 10 mmHg higher than that of plasma.

CSF is produced by the choroid plexus around blood vessels in the lateral ventricles as well as in the walls of the third and fourth ventricles.

Normal lumbar CSF pressure is between 7 and 18 cmCSF. The pH of CSF is 7.33.

36 **A** = True   **B** = True   **C** = True   **D** = False   **E** = False   **F** = True

The anterolateral spinothalamic tract carries information of contralateral touch, nociception and temperature. In general, but not exclusively, the anterior spinothalamic tract conveys touch and the lateral one conveys information about noxious stimuli and temperature.

Fibres that signal proprioception and fine touch run in the ascending dorsal (posterior) columns to the gracile and cuneate nuclei in the medulla. After synapsing there, the second-order fibres decussate to project in the medial lemniscal pathway to the ventral posterior nucleus of the thalamus.

In the dorsal column pathway, the sacral and lumbar fibres lie medial to the thoracic and cervical fibres. In the spinothalamic tract, the sacral and lumbar fibres are displaced more laterally to the thoracic and cervical fibres. It is important to remember this when diagnosing extrinsic and intrinsic spinal tumours causing spinal compression.

The descending corticospinal tract largely decussates at the medullary pyramids and 80% is from then on known as the lateral corticospinal tract that synapses with anterior horn cells to innervate distal limb musculature. Approximately 20% of the corticospinal tract does not decussate at the medulla and continues as the anterior corticospinal tract. This tract plays an important role in controlling the truncal limb musculature.

The Babinski sign is a dorsiflexion response of the toes along with some fanning on scratching the outer aspects of the sole of the foot. In a normal individual the response should be plantarflexion due to control by the lateral corticospinal tract. The Babinski sign indicates damage to the lateral corticospinal tract, but its true significance is not clear.

37 **A** = False **B** = True **C** = True **D** = True **E** = False

The knee and ankle jerks are examples of monosynaptic stretch reflexes elicited by stretch of intrafusal muscle spindle fibres.

A direct synapse on to the ipsilateral α-motor neurone innervating the regular contracting extrafusal muscle fibres causes muscle contraction. The muscle spindles lie parallel to the rest of the muscle fibres and reduce firing when the extrafusal fibres contract.

During fine motor control γ-motor innervation of the intrafusal spindle fibres allows the muscle spindle to discharge and remain sensitive throughout muscle contraction. This becomes a polysynaptic pathway of feedback control and is described as 'α-γ co-activation'.

Golgi tendon organs are sensory nerve endings amongst tendon fascicles that are in series with muscle fibres. They are therefore stimulated by anything that produces tension in the muscle (passive stretch and active muscle contraction). They regulate muscle force and form part of a protective reflex arc. The afferent fibres from the Golgi tendon organs synapse on to spinal cord inhibitory interneurones that synapse on to the muscle motor neurone to cause inhibition. Excitatory innervation of antagonists may also be seen. This reflex is at least disynaptic.

38 **A** = False **B** = False **C** = True **D** = False **E** = False **F** = False

The cerebellum has three functional parts:

1 The ipsilateral nodulus (on the vermis) and the flocculus form, the flocculonodular lobe (vestibulocerebellum). This receives vestibular afferent input and is involved in equilibrium.
2 The remainder of the vermis and the medial hemispheres form the spinocerebellum

and receive proprioceptive afferent input from the ipsilateral body as well as afferent input from the motor cortex. It is important in feedback coordination of movements and action.

3 The lateral hemispheres are called the neocerebellum and these interact with the motor cortex in planning and programming motor commands.

It is worth noting that the mid-line cerebellum controls axial and proximal limb muscles and lesions result in truncal ataxia, whereas the lateral hemispheres control distal muscles and lesions result in distal ataxia. Lesions of the motor cortex must involve deep nuclei to produce ataxia.

In cerebellar lesions, stretch reflexes such as the knee jerk become hypotonic. Cerebellar lesions are generally manifest with movement. Tremor is not seen at rest, but during voluntary work (intention tremor).

Ocular physiology

The tears

39 **A** = True   **B** = False   **C** = False   **D** = True   **E** = False

Lacrimal secretion contains four principal antibacterial proteins: lysozyme, a low molecular weight enzyme that attacks bacterial cell walls, betalysin, lactoferrin, an iron binding protein that also has free radical scavenger properties, and secretary immunoglobulin A (IgA).

Aqueous tear production decreases with age. However, it is asymptomatic until a critical level is reached. Basal tear production is 1.2 ml/min.

The mucin layer is a two-layer structure with an inner tight glycocalyx secreted by corneal epithelial cells, and a looser outer 'mucus blanket' produced by palpebral and bulbar conjunctiva goblet cells. The cornea has no goblet cells.

40 **A** = True   **B** = True   **C** = False   **D** = True   **E** = False

Pre-corneal tear film is made of three layers: lipid, aqueous and mucin layers, with a thickness of up to 10 μm. The outer lipid layer is produced mainly by the meibomian glands of the upper and lower eyelids, with a small component from the glands of Zeiss and Moll. The aqueous layer forms 90% of the thickness of the tear film and is usually slightly hypotonic. Tears are predominantly produced by the orbital and palpebral parts of the main lacrimal gland, and small amounts are produced by accessory glands of Krause and Wolfring. All aqueous production is stimulus driven and is seen to decrease during sleep and general anaesthesia. The lacrimal gland is a tubuloacinar gland with granular acinar cells forming around 80% of the gland's substance. It produces serous fluid and a small amount of mucus.

41 **A** = False   **B** = True   **C** = False   **D** = True   **E** = True

In order for the lipid layer of the tear film to be liquid at ocular surface temperature, properties of meibum include a lower melting temperature than normal skin sebaceous secretion.

Three-quarters of tear volume is eliminated by the lacrimal drainage system, one-quarter is evaporated. Of that drained, two-thirds is drained by the lower canaliculus and one-third by the upper canaliculus.

The majority of oxygen used by the cornea is derived by diffusion from the tear film and not from the anterior chamber. In view of the above figures, it is clear that contact lenses of low oxygen permeability can reduce oxygen availability below critical levels, causing epithelial and stromal oedema along with endothelial changes.

The eyelids

42 **A** = False   **B** = False   **C** = False   **D** = True   **E** = True

The eyelids are made up of six layers: skin, subcutaneous tissue, obicularis, submuscular connective tissue (containing vessels and nerves), fibrous tarsal plate and the palpebral conjunctiva.

Cilia are normally replaced every 3–5 months, but are replaced in two months if forcibly removed.

Bell's phenomenon is the upward rotation of the globe during forced closure of the eyelid, that is, when the patient is asked to close his eyes whilst the eyelids are held open. The A-P axis rotates 15° above the horizontal. It is not seen in reflex blink closure, where there is rotation of 1–2° towards the primary direction of gaze, and approximately 1 mm retraction of the globe. Bell's phenomenon is absent in 10% of the population. The excitability of a nerve can be described by the weakest stimulus that elicits an action potential if applied for an infinite time. This is known as the rheobase. Chronaxie is defined as the time taken to elicit an action potential if a current twice the rheobase is applied. Chronaxie is a measure of excitability of a muscle. The palpebral portion of obicularis oculi has a chronaxie half that of the orbital portion.

Spontaneous blinking is blinking occurring on a regular basis without an apparent external stimulus. It is constant for an individual in a specific environment, but may change with visual acuity, increase with emotional stress, dry air and wind and decrease in rate during stressful visual tasks and with alcohol. It is absent until the third month of life, and some suggest that men and women have similar rates.

43 **A** = True   **B** = False   **C** = False   **D** = True   **E** = True

Corneal blink reflex consists of an ipsilateral disynaptic fast phase with a latency of 10–15 ms and a second slower bilateral multisynaptic phase with a 20–35 ms latency and a poorly understood fast multisynaptic bilateral phase. Pathways involved include the ipsilateral trigeminal nucleus, the pontomedullary 'blink' premotor areas (superior colliculus, red nucleus and pretectal nucleus) and finally the facial nucleus. There are also imputs from the cortex and cerebellum, linking coordination, behaviour and learnt responses.

Due to its high elasticity and loose connection to the underlying muscle, the dermis or corium of the skin of the eyelid is easily distended by oedema or haematoma that commonly collects here and lifts it away from the underlying orbicularis muscle.

An average of two glands of Zeiss empty into each follicle. The modified apocrine sweat glands of Moll are less plentiful and average less than one per follicle. In contrast to the glands of Zeiss, the glands of Moll have no definite function. They may be considered analogous to the pheromone-producing apocrine glands of the axilla.

The conjunctiva consist largely of non-keratinized stratified columnar epithelium except at the limbus and the mucocutaneous junction where it is non-keratinized stratified squamous epithelium. Müller's muscle is better developed in the upper rather than the lower lid, where it attaches to the lower border of the tarsus and is thought to be merely a fibrous extension of the inferior rectus sheath.

44 **A** = True   **B** = False   **C** = False   **D** = False   **E** = False

Myokymia (fibrillary twitching of the eyelids) is seen commonly due to irritation within the VII cranial nerve. It is often idiopathic, but is associated with fatigue, thyrotoxicosis, stress and refractive errors.

The skin layer of the eyelid is the thinnest of the body and contains fine, microscopic lanugo hair. The 100–150 cilia of the upper lid and 50–75 cilia of the lower lid are innervated at their follicles by a neural plexus and have an extremely low threshold for tactile sensation.

At photopic levels, blinking of up to 3 ms duration shows no discontinuity of visual perception.

The sebaceous glands of Zeiss have short, wide ducts lined with stratified squamous epithelium that empty into follicles. They produce sebum from the degeneration of slowly proliferating basal cells and serve to lubricate the eyelashes and prevent them from becoming dry and brittle.

Cornea

45 **A** = False   **B** = True   **C** = False   **D** = True   **E** = True

With eyes closed during sleep, the palpebral conjunctiva (usually superior) is responsible for oxygen delivery to the cornea.

Symptoms of epithelial oedema include 'haloes' and 'rainbows', increased glare sensitivity and decreased contrast sensitivity.

The centre of the cornea is the most sensitive area of the eye, followed by the corneal periphery, the eyelids, the caruncle and the conjunctiva.

'Hassal–Henle warts' are the product of excess basal lamina material produced by the corneal endothelium and are common up to the edge of the corneoscleral limbus. In the centre they are known as guttata.

46 **A** = True   **B** = False   **C** = False   **D** = False   **E** = True

Normal healthy corneal endothelium consists of up to 80% hexagonal cells. Any decrease in this level (an increase of different shapes cells) is known as pleomorphism and can indicate endothelial instability or stress.

Corneal 'temperature reversal' describes how the cornea maintains its hydration and thickness by a metabolically active process that is impaired and allows swelling as surrounding temperature falls. Transendothelial potential is 0.5 mV (500 μV). It is maintained by a basolateral Na^+K^+ ATPase pump, basolateral amiloride-sensitive Na^+/H^+ exchange, and energy-dependent apical Na^+/HCO_3^- transport. Although *in vitro* studies with carbonic anhydrase inhibitors have shown corneal swelling, acetazolamide has shown no effect on corneal hydration.

Aqueous sodium concentration is 143 mmol/l and the stromal sodium concentration is approximately 160–170 mmol/l. However, due to binding with negatively charged glycosaminoglycans, the activity of sodium in the stroma is reduced to 134 mEq/l.

The difference between mmol/l and mEq/l relates to the presence of charged particles. One equivalent (Eq) is 1 mol of an ionized substance divided by its valency.

47 **A** = False   **B** = False   **C** = True   **D** = True   **E** = False   **F** = True

The corneal stroma consists of 78% water or 3.45 parts weight of water to one part solid. As its hydration increases, the ability to swell decreases. The force needed to prevent stromal swelling, also known as swelling pressure, decreases almost exponentially with increasing stromal hydration and thickness. The normal value of swelling pressure is approximately 55 mmHg. Water entering the stroma is influenced by negatively charged glycosaminoglycans and fluid viscosity. Water leaving the stroma is due to the 'endothelial pump' mechanism and an established osmotic gradient.

Evaporation occurs during the day whilst the eyes are open, and it is noted that corneal oedema is greater in the mornings due to a lack of nocturnal evaporation.

In response to stromal wounding, polymorphonuclear leukocytes and then macrophages may appear and fibroblast transformation is seen. Stromal keratocytes hypertrophy and proliferate before reforming and reconnecting gap junctions. Tensile strength may take years to improve. Central corneal injuries heal slower than peripheral wounds.

48 **A** = False   **B** = False   **C** = True   **D** = False   **E** = True   **F** = True

Immediate events after corneal abrasion include a cessation of mitosis and loss of hemidesmosomal attachment of cells at the wound edge to the underlying basement membrane. This allows cells to enlarge to some degree (increase cell water content) and migrate at a rapid rate over any epithelial defect. Mitosis then resumes after wound closure. Cell movement is dependent on calcium calmodulin and cAMP. The effect of cholera toxin is to prevent breakdown of cAMP.

The outer membrane of the superficial cell layer accounts for 60% of total corneal resistance to ion flow due to high paracellular resistance. A transepithelial potential of between 10 and 35 mV exists. It is the difference between stromal potential and tear potential.

Chloride (Cl^-) transport into the epithelium is dependent on secondary active co-transport (linked to the sodium gradient) from the stroma and passive diffusion along the concentration gradient to the tears, regulated by cAMP. The sodium gradient is created by the ubiquitous Na^+K^+ ATPase pump on the basolateral membrane.

Due to an intact barrier formed by junctional complexes, the normal corneal epithelial surface is impermeable to fluorescein dye and stains very little or not at all with this anionic molecule.

49 **A** = False   **B** = True   **C** = True   **D** = False   **E** = True

The cornea is made up of five layers: epithelium, Bowman's membranes, stroma, Descemet's membrane and endothelium. It transmits radiation from 310 nm (in UV) to 2500 nm (infrared). It is most sensitive to UV radiation at 270 nm which can result in photokeratitis.

Corneal epithelial wing cells contain abundant intracellular tonofilaments made up of keratin subunits. They are rich in 64 kD a keratin specific to corneal epithelium. However, the corneal epithelium is non-keratinized because it is unlike the cornified structure of the skin epithelium. In vitamin A deficiency, the corneal epithelium expresses keratins normally found in skin epidermis (xerophthalmia).

Corneal epithelial turnover is within 7 days (once a week).

Corneal epithelium consists of a basal layer forming a single layer of cuboidal cells, over which lie 2–3 layers of wing-shaped cells, and a final outermost, terminally differentiated, degenerating, irregular polygonal superficial layer of cells covered with a dense coat of microvilli.

Collagen forms 71% of the dry weight of the corneal stroma and is mainly type I. There are, however, lesser amounts of type III, type IV, type V and type VI collagen also present.

50 **A** = False   **B** = True   **C** = False   **D** = True   **E** = True

Corneal endothelium is a single layer of non-vascular cells with a high metabolic activity. Although aerobic metabolism in the form of the pentose phosphate shunt system and Krebs cycle is present in the corneal epithelium, stroma and endothelium, the cornea derives most of its energy from anaerobic metabolism. Over three-quarters of glucose is metabolized to lactate which either diffuses slowly across the stroma and endothelium into the aqueous, or is metabolized via the Embden–Meyerhoff pathway in the stroma.

The anterior surface of the cornea is the major refractive surface of the eye, providing 48 dioptres. Posterior surface provides −5 dioptres.

The precorneal tear film possesses an inner mucin layer which partly consists of a glycocalyx (known as the buffy coat) that interacts with the thick layer of microvilli projecting from the superficial cells of the corneal epithelium.

Endothelial cell density at birth is approximately 3500–4000 cells/mm^2. The adult cornea has a cell density between 1400 and 2500 cells/mm^2. Corneal transplants may have less than 1000 cells/mm^2 and still remain clear with normal functions. The critical level for adequate corneal function is between 400 and 700 cells/mm^2 approximately.

51 **A** = False   **B** = True   **C** = False   **D** = False   **E** = True

Bowman's layer is an acellular structureless layer that, when viewed under electron microscopy, can be seen to consist of randomly arranged collagen fibril. It has a thickness of 12 μm and so is approximately one-fifth of the 50–60 μm thick corneal epithelium. The basement membrane of the corneal epithelium consists mainly of type VII collagen known as anchoring fibrils which penetrate into the stroma in order to anchor the overlying basal cells. Type IV collagen exists, however, only in the periphery.

The stroma makes up 90% of the corneal thickness. Descemet's membrane has a thickness of 10–15 μm.

52 **A** = False   **B** = True   **C** = True   **D** = False   **E** = True

Long-term contact lens use is associated with pleomorphism (change in endothelial cell shape) and polymegathism (change in cell size). However, cell loss has not been observed.

Descemet's membrane is 10–15 μm thick and consists of two layers: an anterior layer, which is fetal in origin, and the posterior layer, which is secreted by the endothelium and increases in thickness throughout life. Due to Descemet's membrane having a high resistance to proteolytic enzymes and degradation, it can remain intact even in the presence of severe corneal ulceration.

Endothelial cells possess tight junctions in deep layers, but are also interconnected by gap junctions and act as a relatively leaky barrier between aqueous humour and stroma. Control of corneal hydration is dependent on an active 'endothelial pump' mechanism.

It has been observed that corneal denervation increases the risk of corneal erosion and ulceration (neurotrophic). The absence of implicated neuropeptides such as substance P and CGRP from corneal nerve terminals has a delaying effect on corneal wound healing.

53 **A** = True   **B** = True   **C** = True   **D** = False   **E** = True   **F** = False

The stromal plexus of myelinated and unmyelinated axons enter radially into the cornea at the limbus and within 1 mm become unmyelinated whilst retaining a Schwann cell covering.

Collagen fibrils of the stroma have a diameter of 24–30 nm and a lamellar arrangement with a macroperiodicity of 64 nm.

Corneal sensitivity is up to four times greater in blue-eyed individuals than in those with brown eyes. Albinos with an absence of pigment show a reduced sensitivity. There is no explanation for this observation.

The corneal epithelium has pain and cold receptors as well as chemical receptors for low pH and hypertonic solutions. This information is carried by Aδ fibres.

Although measurement of endothelial cell density is useful in assessing corneal endothelium stability, it must be measured alongside endothelial cell size and shape. The size is measured by the area of the apical surface of a cell population. From repeated calculations, mean cell size and standard deviations can be derived. An increase/decrease in size is known as polymegathism. For a given cell density, there may be widely varying degrees of polymegathism and pleomorphism.

Aqueous and ciliary epithelium

54 **A** = False   **B** = False   **C** = True   **D** = False   **E** = False

Aqueous production is between 2 and 2.5 μl/min.

The non-pigmented ciliary epithelium plays the major role in aqueous formation due to the presence of active enzyme systems in the clefts, including the Na$^+$K$^+$ ATPase, carbonic anhydrase and adenylate cyclase. Active secretion accounts for over 70% of aqueous production with ultrafiltration producing up to 15% and passive diffusion largely accounting for the remainder. Aqueous flow decreases by up to 40% during sleep.

The corneal endothelium pumps fluid into the anterior chamber at a rate of 10 μl/h. This amounts to approximately 8% of the aqueous production rate.

55 **A** = True   **B** = False   **C** = False   **D** = False   **E** = False

The main pathway for aqueous outflow is via the pressure- and resistance-dependent trabecular meshwork pathway. Valsalva manoeuvre increases the central venous pressure, episcleral venous pressure and reduces outflow, causing intraocular pressure to rise.

The pressure-independent uveoscleral outflow of aqueous appears to show no evidence of an active process.

Intraocular pressure in the general population does not fit the bell-shaped normal Gaussian distribution. There is a greater distribution of the population with higher pressures. It is said to be 'skewed' to the right. Strenuous exercise can briefly lower intraocular pressure, perhaps due to metabolic changes, such as acidosis or extra-cellular fluid volume changes. Inspiration causes an increase in negative intrapleural pressure. This reduces central venous pressure, allowing increased venous return to the heart. Reduced central venous pressure reduces episcleral venous pressure and increases outflow of the aqueous. Inspiration is thus seen to cause a brief fall in intraocular pressure. Valsalva manoeuvre however, causes a positive intrapleural pressure and increases central venous pressure. The result is a rise in intraocular pressure.

56 **A** = True   **B** = False   **C** = False   **D** = True   **E** = False

Small quantities of complement C2, C6 and C7 are found in normal (primary) aqueous. The trabecular meshwork is divided into an inner uveal layer, a corneoscleral layer and an outer juxtacanalicular layer of endothelial cells. The juxtacanalicular layer offers most resistance to aqueous outflow. The aqueous enters these endothelial cells and by a process of vacuolation is exocytosed into Schlemm's canal.

The uveoscleral drainage of aqueous reaches the suprachoroidal space and either passes across the sclera or follows the large vessels piercing the sclera.

The pulsatile nature of intraocular pressure is due to the pulsatile arterial ocular blood flow of the choroidal circulation, which is much larger than the central retinal artery circulation.

57 **A** = False   **B** = True   **C** = False   **D** = True   **E** = False

IgG is the only detectable immunoglobulin in the aqueous. IgA and IgM are found to be present in conditions such as uveitis where there is breakdown of the blood–aqueous barrier.

Plasma protein concentration is of the order of 6–7 g/100 ml. Aqueous protein concentration is between 5 and 15 mg/100 ml in humans. Of the coagulation/fibrinolytic proteins, only plasminogen and plasminogen proactivator are found in significant amounts in the aqueous. Insulin levels in the aqueous are 3% of those in plasma and increase by a factor of 10 postprandially.

Although active aqueous secretion is independent of changes in intraocular pressure, it is however, found to decrease sharply with intraocular pressures greater than 50–60 mmHg, approaching that of ciliary artery pressure.

58 **A** = True   **B** = True   **C** = False   **D** = False   **E** = True

Water-soluble substances such as glucose, amino acids and metabolic substrates cross the blood–aqueous barrier by carrier-mediated transport. Aqueous production and intraocular pressure have a diurnal variation with a peak between 7 and 9 am.

The rate of aqueous production has been found to fall with age.

Glucose concentration in CSF is approximately two-thirds that of plasma. Concentration of glucose in aqueous is 80% of that in plasma.

59 **A** = False **B** = True **C** = True **D** = True **E** = True

The blood–aqueous barrier is formed by apical tight junctions of the non-pigmented ciliary epithelial cells and by the tight junctions between the capillary endothelial cells of the non-fenestrated iris vessels. Urea passes slowly across the blood–aqueous barrier and is excreted slowly by the kidney. It is more effective than mannitol in acutely reducing intraocular pressure. Urea causes local complications of phlebitis and sloughing as well as systemic complications, and therefore the use of mannitol is considered more effective and popular.

60 **A** = False **B** = True **C** = True **D** = False **E** = False

The ciliary body is made up of a smooth pars plana posteriorly and a pars plicata anteriorly. The apical aspects of the pigmented ciliary epithelial cell faces the apical aspect of the non-pigmented epithelial cells.

Tight junctions exist between the apices of the inner non-pigmented ciliary epithelial cells. Gap junctions exist between pigmented ciliary epithelial cells and also between pigmented and non-pigmented ciliary epithelial cells. Capillaries of the ciliary body are fenestrated and thin walled, whereas those of the liver sinusoids are discontinuous, allowing easy passage of blood cells through capillary walls.

61 **A** = False **B** = True **C** = True **D** = False **E** = True

In the mature eye pigmented epithelial cells are cuboidal and non-pigmented cells are columnar. By inhibiting carbonic anhydrase and the synthesis of bicarbonate, acetazolamide has been found to reduce aqueous production by up to 50%.

Ciliary epithelia secrete primary aqueous humour. Secondary aqueous humour refers to the leakage of plasma-like (or plasmoid) aqueous through destabilization of the blood–aqueous barrier. Prostaglandins E and F disrupt the apical tight junctions of the non-pigmented epithelial cells.

Pupil

62 **A** = False **B** = True **C** = False **D** = True **E** = False

Pupil diameter can range from 1 mm to 9 mm when fully dilated. Pupil size gradually decreases with age, but is largest in adolescence. It is common to have unequal pupil sizes, and simply physiological anisocoria is present in 20% of the population. It is not constant in an individual and can increase, decrease, or reverse sides in a matter of hours. In the presence of unequal pupils the reaction to changes in light and accommodation are of crucial importance.

The reaction to light has a relatively long latent period that is expected with smooth muscle. In bright light it is 0.2 s and in dimmed light it is prolonged up to 0.5 s.

A tonic pupil is one of the many causes of an efferent pupillary defect, where the pupil reacts poorly to light and appears fixed and dilated. It refers to any postganglionic parasympathetic denervation of the intraocular muscles, and implies damage to the ciliary ganglion or short ciliary nerves by orbital trauma, viral infection, neoplasm or other causes.

Although damage to the third nerve by space-occupying lesion can cause an efferent pupillary defect, it is not referred to as a tonic pupil.

63 **A** = True   **B** = True   **C** = True   **D** = False   **E** = True

Following pupillary dilation, patients experience blurred vision due to spherical aberrations highlighted by the large pupil aperture. Furthermore, accommodation may be impaired with the use of cycloplegic drugs.

Pupillary dilation is a therapeutic procedure in cases of anterior uveitis in order to prevent synechiae and ciliary spasm.

Cycloplegic mydriatics carry a risk of raising intraocular pressure, especially in long-term use.

64 **A** = True   **B** = True   **C** = True   **D** = True   **E** = True

Factors influencing the size of a pupil may be categorized into mechanical, extrinsic and intrinsic factors. Sphincter pupillae has a stronger influence than dilater pupillae on pupil size. Mechanical factors include iris pigment. A brown iris is associated with a smaller pupil than a blue iris. Lesions to the iris musculature also affect pupil size and shape.

Extrinsic factors include light or dark adaptation, distance of the object of fixation and the degree of change in illumination presented to the retina.

Intrinsic factors include sympathetic tone causing mydriasis, parasympathetic tone causing miosis, age, emotion and sleep.

Sleep, fatigue and drowsiness are associated with reduced sympathetic tone and reduced inhibition of the Edinger–Westphal nucleus, causing miosis.

65 **A** = False   **B** = True   **C** = True   **D** = False   **E** = False

Dense lens opacities do not cause afferent pupillary defects. An efferent pupillary defect describes a fixed dilated pupil and can be caused by any defect in the pathway of the mid-brain (third cranial nerve, ciliary ganglion) to the iris. It may also be caused by mydriatic drugs, including anticholinergic or adrenergic agents.

Adie's tonic pupil is an idiopathic tonic pupil associated with benign tendon are-flexia. Pupillary response to light is poor, but pupillary response to near vision is strong and tonic with delayed accommodation of distant objects and symptoms of blurred vision. It is suggested that these strong pupillary responses to near vision may be due to aberrant regenerating nerve fibres from the ciliary muscle to the constrictor pupillae muscle. Cholinergic hypersensitivity is seen, implying a defect in the ciliary ganglion. The condition usually affects young women unilaterally, but may become bilateral.

Argyll-Robertson pupils describe lesions to the relay paths in the tectum between afferent and efferent tracks. It was originally associated with tabes dorsalis. In distinc-tion to the Adie's pupil, the pupils are small (spinal miosis) and the accommodation reflex is preserved (Argyll-Robertson Pupil = Accommodation Reflex Preserved). Whereas a tonic pupil dilates well with atropine, Argyll-Robertson pupils dilate poorly.

66 **A** = True   **B** = False   **C** = False   **D** = False   **E** = True

Botulinum toxin blocks the release of acetylcholine at both preganglionic and post-ganglionic levels. Atropine is a competitive antimuscarinic antagonist of acetylcholine at the post synaptic cell membrane. Reversible acetylcholine esterase inhibitors such as pyridostigmine (mesthinon), edrophonium (tensilon), neostigmine and physostigmine (eserine) cause miosis by potentiating acetylcholine.

Drugs such as noradrenaline, adrenaline, phenylephrine and methoxamine are direct α-adrenergic agonists causing mydriasis without cycloplegia. They do not affect the pupillary light reflex or accommodation.

Central nervous system depressants such as barbituates (phenobarbitone) act by the GABA system to potentiate neural inhibition of the Edinger–Westphal nucleus. Barbi-turate poisoning results in sluggish pupillary light reflexes.

67 **A** = True   **B** = True   **C** = True   **D** = False   **E** = True

Histamine acts directly on smooth muscle causing it to contract. As sphincter pupillae is stronger than dilator pupillae, the result is a powerful miosis.

Morphine acting directly on smooth muscle causes constriction, and so its direct action on sphincter pupillae results in miosis. The classical pinpoint pupil seen mor-phine overdose, however, is probably due to central nervous system depression and so reduced cortical inhibition of the Edinger–Westphal nucleus.

Pilocarpine is a complex rather than simple direct acting muscarinic cholinergic agonist. As well as causing miosis, it has a puzzling effect of reducing, or even abolishing the pupillary light reflex for many hours after miosis disappears, thus coun-teracting naturally released acetylcholine.

Cocaine causes mydriasis by preventing reuptake of noradrenaline back into nerve terminals. Its duration is variable and no rebound miosis is seen. It also causes anaesthesia and vasoconstriction that results in conjunctival blanching.

Thymoxamine is a competitive α-adrenergic antagonist and causes miosis. It reverses phenylephrine and hydroxyamphetamine mydriasis. It does not reverse mydriasis of anticholenergic drugs, and has no apparent affect on the ciliary body and thus accommodation.

68 **A** = True **B** = True **C** = False **D** = False **E** = False

Johann Friedrich Horner described a case report of a preganglionic lesion in 1869. The sympathetic pathway can be divided into a central, preganglionic and postganglionic parts, and this forms a classification of the aetiology of Horner's syndrome. Clinical signs include ptosis, miosis, facial anhydrosis (in preganglionic Horner's), dilation lag and, initially, conjunctival hyperaemia may be seen. Congenital or neonatal Horner's denies normal pigmentation of the iris. Horner's after the age of 2 years usually does not cause heterochromia.

Cocaine prevents reuptake of noradrenaline and any interruption in the sympathetic pathway will reduce the noradrenaline released from nerve endings. As a rule, therefore, cocaine dilation is reduced in all Horner's pupils.

Based on the principle of denervation hypersensitivity, postganglionic Horner's pupils can dilate with low concentrations of adrenaline.

Pancoast's syndrome describes lung carcinoma associated with ipsilateral preganglionic Horner's syndrome due to invasion of the cervical sympathetic plexus in the region of the stellate ganglion. Hydroxyamphetamine is an indirect α-adrenergic agonist that only dilates the pupil in the presence of presynaptic noradrenaline. It therefore produces mydriasis in central and preganglionic Horner's, but fails to dilate the eye in lesions of the postganglionic sympathetic pathway. The hydroxyamphetamine test is said to have a diagnostic accuracy of 84% for postganglionic lesions and 97% for central or preganglionic lesions.

The lens

69 **A** = False **B** = True **C** = True **D** = False **E** = False

The lens absorbs short-wave length blue/ultraviolet light.

The acellular capsule is analogous to basement membrane. It stains positive with PAS reagents. It is therefore probably the thickest basement membrane in the body and is made up of type IV collagen and 10% glycosaminoglycan. It is synthesized by the epithelium and the most superficial lens fibres posteriorly.

Compared to other tissue, the lens is unique in being made up of one-third protein and two-thirds water. This high protein content is thought to be essential for the high refractive index, and also affords a good buffering capacity. The pH of the lens has been measured at 6.9.

Lens proteins have very little helical structure. Crystallin configuration is mainly β-sheet. The fibres of the lens are closely packed with a distance of 100/200 Å between adjacent cells. Lens transparency is thought to be achieved by the close packing (reducing light scattering), the regular arrangement and the small differences in refracted index between light-scattering components.

70 **A** = True   **B** = True   **C** = False   **D** = True   **E** = False

In the lens, a potassium concentration of 125 mmol/l and a sodium concentration of 20 mmol/l is maintained by the Na⁺K⁺ ATPase pump actively pumping sodium out and potassium in.

Of the extremely high 33% protein content of the lens, 90% are water-soluble structural proteins or crystallins.

Glutathione, a tripeptide, is present in the lens in concentrations 1000 times greater than that of the aqueous. It is continually synthesized and maintained in its reduced form (GSH) by NADPH from the hexose monophosphate (HMP) shunt. In the presence of cataract, glutathione levels are found to be reduced.

71 **A** = False   **B** = True   **C** = True   **D** = False   **E** = True

Central lens epithelial cells are cuboidal. At the equator they elongate and differentiate into lens fibres. Functions of the lens epithelial cells include cell division, especially in the equatorial and pre-equatorial regions, synthesis of crystallin proteins, active cation transport and secretion of the capsule.

Lens fibre nuclei are lost at the deep cortical/nuclear stage. Nucleated lens fibre cells containing organelles are usually 'hidden' behind the iris and not in the optical path.

The Na⁺K⁺ ATPase pump is mainly found on the apicolateral surface of the lens epithelium.

The lens interior has an osmolality similar to that of aqueous humour.

72 **A** = True   **B** = True   **C** = True   **D** = True   **E** = True

Insulin levels in the aqueous humour are 3% of that in serum. The lens has insulin receptors, although glucose enters the lens by insulin-independent facilitated diffusion.

Although 80% of lens glucose is metabolized by anaerobic glycolysis, and 4% is metabolized by aerobic glycolysis, due to a yield of two ATP molecules per glucose molecule, anaerobic glycolysis produces 60% of lens energy and aerobic glycolysis produces up to 40% of lens energy (yielding 36 ATP per glucose molecule). Ffiteen per cent of glucose is metabolized via the pentose (HMP) shunt.

Active transport mechanisms of amino acids into the lens are dependent on the sodium gradient set up by the Na^+K^+ ATPase pump.

The sorbitol pathway serves as a protective buffer that can reduce hypertonicity of the lens due to high glucose levels in the aqueous as a result of short-term hyperglycaemia. This is based on the observation that a rapid rise is in serum glucose (i.e. 5–15 mM) can markedly dehydrate the lens. Excess glucose is converted to sorbitol and then to fructose which diffuses out of the lens.

In 1978, Stevens *et al.* put forward the proposal that sustained activity of the sorbitol pathway in diabetes was not the major cause of diabetic cataract. It was suggested that glycosylation of lens proteins was the cause. Calcium levels in the lens are of the order of 0.3 mEq/kg lens water. Efflux of Ca^{2+} is an active process independent of Na^+–Ca^{2+} exchange or external levels of Na^+. The mechanism may due to a Ca^{2+} ATPase pump.

73 A = True   **B** = True   **C** = False   **D** = True   **E** = False

Alpha, beta and gamma crystallins are the only crystallins found in humans. Alpha crystallin has been found in the heart, brain and lung. Alpha crystallins are related to 'heat shock' proteins, protective proteins that bind any denatured proteins made in response to unusual rises in temperature.

Alpha crystallin is the largest crystallin and is mainly found in the cortex. It comprises of 35% of lens crystallins. Beta crystallin is the most common crystallin, making up 55% of lens crystallins. Gamma crystallin forms 10% of lens crystallins. It is the smallest crystallin and is monomeric, unlike the others. Gamma crystallins are found mainly at the central core region, the fetal nucleus of the lens. It is the area of highest refractive index and the lowest water content of the lens. Due to very low protein turnover here, the lifetime of the gamma crystallin molecule is the same as that of the mammal. Due to cysteine-, methionine- and sulphur-containing residues, it is susceptible to oxidative processes and nuclear cataract formation.

74 A = True   **B** = False   **C** = True   **D** = True   **E** = True

A cataract is usually defined as an opacification of the lens. Increased levels of lens calcium is associated with deposits of calcium oxalate and cortical cataracts. Hypocalcaemia (as a result of hypoparathyroidism) is also associated with outer cortical lens opacification. Other metabolic disorders that cause cataract include diabetes, galactosaemia, Wilson's disease and homocystinuria.

In cataract, both methionine and cysteine are found to be oxidized.

Photosensitizing drugs such as psoralen given in combination with brief exposures to UV radiation (320–340 nm) are able to photochemically change and modify nearby tissue molecules. PUVA is widely used by dermatologists to treat psoriasis. The most commonly affected tissues are the skin and the eye. Formation of cataracts is well documented.

The mechanism for steroid-induced cataract is unclear and amongst many theories Urban and Cotlier (1986) proposed that steroids react with amino groups of lens crystallins to precipitate the formation of disulphide bonds leading to protein aggregation. Posterior subcapsular cataracts are commonly caused by topical and systemic corticosteroid. Chlorpromazine is the only phenothiazine implicated in causing cataract.

75 **A** = True   **B** = True   **C** = True   **D** = False   **E** = True

The lens is insensitive to touch or pain due to the absence of sensory innervation. Increase of thickness and also equatorial growth of the human lens occurs at approximately 0.02 mm per year. The variation in the anterior radius of curvature is between 8.4 and 13.8 mm with an average of 10 mm. The posterior radius of curvature is between 4.6 and 7.5 mm with an average of 6 mm. These figures are age related.

During accommodation, the anterior surface of the lens moves forward towards the cornea, and the posterior surface back, but to a much smaller extent than the anterior surface.

The lens capsule continues to grow throughout life and a young adult's capsule measures approximately 13 μm anteriorly and approximately 4 μm posteriorly.

Vitreous

76 **A** = True   **B** = False   **C** = False   **D** = False   **E** = True

Due to a low diffusion gradient, high molecular weight molecules are carried in the vitreous by convective bulk flow.

Hyaluronic acid provides greatest resistance to flow of water in the vitreous, especially in the cortex. Collagen provides resistance to bulk flow.

Hyaluronic acid has an anionic charge which allows it to interact with mobile ions and influence osmotic pressure, ion transport and vitreal electric potential.

Although zonule fibres are similar to vitreous collagen fibrils they differ in certain aspects: they are tightly packed and resist collagenase, whereas vitreous collagen fibres are loosely arranged and are susceptible to collagenase activity.

Liquefaction describes an increase in the liquid volume of the vitreous. Age-related liquefaction of the vitreous begins in the central vitreous and by the age of 50, up to 25% of individuals have a significant degree of liquefaction.

77 **A** = True   **B** = False   **C** = True   **D** = True   **E** = True

Fibroblasts are mainly found in the vitreous base and adjacent to the optic disc and ciliary processes. The vitreous has marked haemostatic properties and has been shown to shorten the partial thromboplastin time and cause platelet aggregation.

The vitreous serves as a repository of nutrients (including amino acids) for the retina. It has been known for over 50 years that the vitreous has active water movement important for transport of solutes in the eye. Fifty per cent of labelled water is seen to turn over every 10–15 min.

78 A = False **B** = True **C** = True **D** = False **E** = True

Collagen density is greatest in the vitreous base, followed by the posterior vitreous cortex and then the anterior vitreous cortex behind the lens.

Cloquet's canal, the former site of the hyaloid artery, is devoid of collagen fibrils and consists of fenestrated sheaths of basal laminae. It opens posteriorly into the optic disc.

The vitreous is made up of 99% water. Hydrated hyaluronic acid has a volume 3000 times greater than when dehydrated. The vitreous is susceptible to osmotic dehydration and reduction in volume from mannitol therapy.

The dense vitreous cortex is absent over the optic disc and is thin over the macula.

Hyalocytes are mononuclear cells found in the region of greatest hyaluronic acid concentration in a single layer anterior to the inner limiting layer of the retina.

79 A = False **B** = False **C** = False **D** = True **E** = False

The vitreous transmits up to 90% of visible light between 300 and 1400 nm. It does not transmit light below 300 nm.

Vitreous osmolality has been measured to range between 288 and 322 mOsm/kg, slightly higher than that of serum.

Due to active pumping of potassium from the aqueous into the lens and then passive diffusion into the anterior vitreous, potassium levels in the vitreous can be used to give an accurate time of death within the first 3–4 days.

Vitreous to plasma ascorbic acid ratio is 9:1, probably due to active ciliary body pumping into the aqueous and then passive diffusion into the vitreous.

80 A = False **B** = True **C** = False **D** = False **E** = True

The vitreous forms 80% of the globe. The refractive index of the vitreous is 1.3349. Collagen is the major structural protein of the vitreous. Over 90% of the collagen is of type II. Collagen and hyaluronic acid are the major structural molecules of the vitreous. In humans, hyaluronic acid content in the vitreous is very low in the prenatal period. Hyalocytes synthesize glycosaminoglycans after birth and maximum levels of vitreous hyaluronic acid are reached by adulthood and are concentrated mainly in the cortex.

81 **A** = False   **B** = True   **C** = False   **D** = True   **E** = True

The central retinal artery receives sympathetic innervation up to the lamina cribrosa and not beyond. Despite this fact, the retinal vessels appear to constrict *in vitro* on exposure to noradrenaline outside the vessel wall. They appear to display both α_1- and α_2-receptors. Sympathetic innervation of the choroidal circulation serves to reduce blood flow by vasoconstriction without affecting the retinal circulation. In this way stable blood flow is maintained during sudden changes in systemic blood pressure. The role of parasympathetic innervation to the retina is unclear. Both retinal and choroidal vessels vasodilate in the presence of hypoxia or hypercapnia (increased P_{CO_2}).

82 **A** = False   **B** = True   **C** = True   **D** = False   **E** = False

Müller cells are a form of ependymal cell. The retina lacks the presence of oligodendrocytes as ganglion cell axons are unmyelinated.

The peak shedding period of cone discs is inconsistent, but shedding of rod discs occurs mainly in the morning.

Evidence suggests that the foveola is deficient in blue cones.

The external limiting membrane is a term referring to the staining of the zonula adherens (intermediate junction) attaching the plasma membranes of photoreceptors and adjacent Müller cells. It separates the photoreceptor layer from the outer nuclear layer.

The central retinal artery is lined with continuous epithelium and supplies the inner two-thirds of the retina, including the inner nuclear layer. The fenestrated choriocapillaris supplies nutrients to the outer third of the retina, including the photoreceptors.

83 **A** = False   **B** = False   **C** = True   **D** = True   **E** = True

Müller cells extend through the entire thickness of the neural retina from the internal limiting membrane to beyond the external limiting membrane, terminating between the inner segments of the photoreceptors.

The ciliary stalk connecting inner and outer segments of the photoreceptor is a modified cilium with nine pairs of microtubules but no central pair.

Rhodopsin lies across the bilayered phospholipid disc membrane. 11-*cis*-Retinaldehyde is bound to opsin by a Schiff-base linkage and only absorbs light that meets it perpendicularly. Light arriving at any other angle is not absorbed. The b-wave of the electroretinogram is a reflection of the potential change in the Müller cell.

84 **A** = False   **B** = True   **C** = True   **D** = True   **E** = False

The Gs protein 'transducin' is made up of three subunits, α, β and γ, and remains inactive due to the presence of the γ subunit.

The retinal pigment epithelium maintains the blood–retinal barrier, phagocytoses photoreceptor outer segments, nutritionally supports the photoreceptors, transports solutes, stores photopigment and absorbs light. The retinal pigment epithelial cells are encircled by zonulae occludentes (tight junctions) as well as zonulae adherentes (inter-mediate junctions) and a few gap junctions on the apicolateral surface.

Retinol enters the retinal pigment epithelium from the bloodstream, assisted by a binding protein. It is immediately esterified to prevent accumulation and toxicity to membranes in the retina. The enzymatic isomerization of the resulting All-*trans*-retinyl ester to 11-*cis*-retinol is followed by oxidation of this product to 11-*cis*-Retinaldehyde. 11-*cis*-Retinaldehyde enters the photoreceptor and binds with opsin to form rhodopsin.

85 **A** = False   **B** = False   **C** = False   **D** = False   **E** = False

cGMP levels are high in the dark and fall on exposure to light due to activation of phosphodiesterase. The 'triad' was first described by Misotten in 1962 and describes the invagination into a cone pedicle of a bipolar cell dendrite flanked by two horizontal cell processes, one on each side.

The retinal pigment epithelium consists of a single layer of cells with a predominantly hexagonal arrangement. Photoreceptor tips are kept in adherence to the retinal pig-ment epithelial processes by the viscous interphotoreceptor matrix. There are no junctional complexes.

86 **A** = False   **B** = False   **C** = False   **D** = True   **E** = True

Rhodopsin has a half-life of 420 years.

The 'dark current' refers to the sodium influx entering the outer segment of the photoreceptor from which it reaches the inner segment via the cytoplasm.

By virtue of the photoreceptor depolarizing to darkness and hyperpolarizing to light, it is an OFF cell.

Approximately 15% of glucose metabolism in the retina is via the hexose monopho-sphate shunt pathway for the production of the reducing substrate NADPH and synth-esis of nucleotides.

The blood flow per gram weight to the retina is up to three times higher than that to the kidney and between 10 and 20 times higher than that to the grey matter of the brain. Oxygen consumption in the retina is twice that of the cerebral cortex.

87 **A** = False   **B** = True   **C** = False   **D** = True   **E** = True

Dietary sources of vitamin A include β-carotene from carrots and sweet potatoes and retinyl esters from animal sources. These are enzymatically converted to retinol, vitamin A alcohol and retinoic acid in the gut.

Conversion of rhodopsin to bathorhodopsin is a photoreaction. Subsequent conversion reactions are thermally driven.

In the dark, the inner segment of the retina, which is supplied by the central retinal artery, is vulnerable to hypoxia due to the high rate of metabolism maintained in the dark current. The choroidal circulation supplies the outer segment and has a high rate of blood flow.

Mitochondria consist of an outer membrane, inner membrane with cristae and a matrix enclosed by the inner membrane. Between the inner and outer membrane is an intermembrane space. The matrix consists of soluble enzymes absent in the cytoplasm. The inner membrane holds electron-transferring proteins and the enzyme ATP synthase. Acetyl CoA is formed from pyruvate by pyruvate dehydrogenase in the matrix.

In the retina, although 60% of glucose is metabolized anaerobically and only 25% is metabolized aerobically, due to its high ATP yield, aerobic metabolism accounts for up to 90% of energy production in the retina. Fifteen per cent of glucose is metabolized by the hexose monophosphate shunt pathway.

88 **A** = False   **B** = True   **C** = True   **D** = True   **E** = False

Photoreceptors are unable to store glycogen. Müller cells store glycogen and are able to convert glycogen to glucose due to the presence of glucose-6-phosphatase.

Terminal processes of ON bipolar cells are found in the inner half of the inner plexiform layer whilst those of OFF bipolar cells are found in the outer half of the inner plexiform layer. These cells are excited by brightness or darkness respectively and they form the beginning of parallel pathways reaching the brain. They are directly excitatory to their specific ganglion cells.

In the retina, pyruvate production (regardless of oxygen supply) is greater than pyruvate metabolism. This causes production of lactate.

Due to the reduced partial pressure of oxygen at high altitude, delayed dark adaptation is seen.

Electrophysiological investigations

89 **A** = True   **B** = True   **C** = True   **D** = True   **E** = False

Electroretinography records the summation of retinal potential changes to light. As the central macula occupies 5% of the photoreceptor population, the ERG may be normal in the presence of severe macular disease. The EOG is able to assess RPE/photoreceptor interaction by recording corneoretinal potentials with fixed 30° lateral excursions. It consists of a standing potential due to RPE activity and a light-sensitive component due to depolarization of the basal membrane of the retinal pigment epithelium. In retinitis pigmentosa the amplitude of the light-sensitive potential falls in early disease and the standing potential is also seen to fall in advanced stages.

Pattern ERG consists of three waves: N35, P50 (partly ganglion cell derived) and N95 (ganglion cell, but secondary phenomenon P50). P50 is abnormal in the presence of macular disease, however the P50/N95 ratio is normal. In the presence of optic neuropathy, P50 is usually normal, but N95 may show selective reduction.

By using monocular stimulation and comparing left and right hemisphere VEPs, the difference in latency and scale distribution between normal and abnormal recordings can be used to predict the location of compressive lesions, as to whether they may be chiasmal, pre- or post-chiasmal. When the retinal is stimulated by a flash of light 10^6 times brighter than that required for scotopic ERG, an early receptor potential is seen to occur before the a-wave. It consists of a positive peak followed by a negative trough and a second positive peak. It is thought to be generated by cone pigments.

90 **A** = False **B** = True **C** = False **D** = False **E** = True

The ERG is a test of the peripheral retina and of cells distal to the ganglion cells. The a-wave of the ERG is produced by photoreceptors which are supplied by the choroidal circulation. Glaucoma is a disease of ganglion cells and the optic nerve and so shows a normal ERG. The flicker ERG produces a pure cone response in the form of a sinusoidal-like wave response. Rods have relatively poor temporal resolution and are unable to respond to flash frequencies greater than 10–15 Hz. The Arden index refers to the light peak/dark trough in the electro-oculogram. The normal value should be greater than 170%. This is a reflection of RPE/photoreceptor interaction.

91 **A** = False **B** = False **C** = True **D** = True **E** = True

The ERG is performed using electrodes placed near the source of the signal close to the cornea. This is achieved with contact lens and non-contact lens corneal electrodes. The VEP is recorded by placing electrodes over the occipital scalp in relation to the visual cortex.

The pattern ERG is useful in detecting ganglion cell abnormalities. It is of no value in confirming central retinal artery occlusion.

The flash VEP uses a diffuse stimulus that is clinically useful in patients not fixating, or those with an unknown refractive error. It has individual variability, but is consistent between cerebral hemispheres and eyes.

The ERG b-wave is largest when the patient is full dark adapted.

The extraocular muscles

92 **A** = False **B** = True **C** = True **D** = False **E** = True

A cross-section of an extraocular muscle such as the rectus, reveals an outer orbital layer, a core and an innermost global layer facing the globe.

Extraocular muscles may be broadly classified into singly innervated fibrillenstrukter fibres and multiply innervated felderstrukter fibres. The fibrillenstrukter fibres are found in the orbital layer, are thought to be responsible for fast speed contraction and have a single large motor end-plate. They have a well-developed sarcoplasmic reticulum and T-tubule system releasing calcium for excitation–contraction coupling. Other varying types are found elsewhere in the muscle with inconsistent features.

The felderstrukter fibres make up most of the core and the global layer of the muscle, although some are found in the orbital aspect as well. These fibres have multiple grape-like nerve endings scattered along their length and are tonically active. Due to a poorly developed sarcoplasmic reticulum, calcium release is from the surface membrane and not the sarcoplasmic reticulum.

The orbital layer of the rectus muscles possesses a richer capillary blood supply and a greater concentration of mitochondria than the global layer.

Sherrington's law of reciprocal innervation states that with increased contraction of a prime mover, there is a decrease in contractile activity of the corresponding antagonist. Yoke muscles are paired muscles that move both eyes in the same direction and are equally innervated (see Hering's law).

Suxamethonium (succinylcholine) initially depolarizes the end-plate and then remains bound causing neuromuscular blockade. It acts rapidly, usually for a short duration (less than 10 min) and is normally hydrolysed by pseudocholinesterases. In the presence of a cholinesterase inhibiter, this breakdown is diminished.

93 **A** = False   **B** = False   **C** = False   **D** = False   **E** = False

Amidst growing arguments against the role of proprioception in extraocular muscles, there do, however, exist three main types of nerve endings which are thought to be sensory. Spiral nerve endings have recently been shown to be motor endings. Scanty muscles spindles with thin capsules and few intrafusal fibres have a questionable role. A few Golgi tendon organs exist, but these are atypical in morphology and also perhaps, in function.

Tertiary positions of gaze involve simultaneous rotations about the X-axis (horizontal) and Z-axis (vertical). Torsion with rotation about the Y-axis is not a tertiary position of gaze. Extorsion and intorsion by inferior and superior obliques respectively involves rotation about a fixed point on the lateral limbus and not about the Y-axis. Secondary positions of gaze involve rotation of the eye along either the vertical Z-axis or the horizontal X-axis.

The isolated agonist model is a well-accepted model of extraocular movement. Medial rectus has a primary action of adduction; lateral rectus: abduction; superior rectus: elevation (secondary action: abduction and intorsion); inferior rectus: depression (secondary action: abduction and extorsion); inferior oblique: extorsion (secondary reaction: abduction and elevation); and superior oblique: intorsion (secondary action: depression and abduction). Due to the insertion of inferior oblique at an angle of 51° to the sagittal plane, it produces pure extorsion when the eye rotates 39° laterally out of the sagittal plane.

PHARMACOLOGY
Questions

1 Complications of periocular injections include

  A transient reduction in visual acuity
  B extraocular muscle palsy
  C central retinal artery occlusion
  D conjunctival haemorrhage
  E glaucoma and cataract

2 Which of the following statements are true?

  A The corneal epithelium acts as a depot for drugs released into the aqueous.
  B The ciliary body provides the largest ocular source of drug-metabolizing enzymes.
  C Topical neomycin can cause blepharoconjunctivitis.
  D Topical timolol can cause bronchospasm, bradycardia and systemic hypotension.
  E Subconjunctival injection is most commonly performed by passing a needle through the skin of the lid between the conjunctiva and Tenon's capsule.

3 Ocular side-effects of digoxin therapy include

  A changes in colour vision after day one of administration
  B impaired dark adaptation
  C reduced intraocular pressure
  D snowy vision
  E retrobulbar neuritis

4 Which of the following statements are correct?

  A β-Adrenergic receptors are found in the corneal epithelium.
  B Topical noradrenaline lowers intraocular pressure mainly by reducing aqueous production.
  C Mydriasis due to topical adrenaline is maximal at 2 h after installation and lasts 12 h.
  D Phenylephrine is a synthetic amine with mainly α-agonist properties.
  E Timolol is administered twice a day.

5 Which of the following are correct?

A Topical adrenaline causes cycloplegia.
B Adrenaline causes maculopathy in aphakic eyes.
C Phenylephrine causes a rebound miosis 24 h after installation.
D Guanethidine blocks the effects of hydroxyamphetamine.
E Pilocarpine, adrenaline and timolol are less effective in reducing intraocular pressure in black subjects than white subjects.

6 Which of the following statements are true?

A One per cent topical adrenaline causes conjunctival blanching, reduction in intraocular pressure and severe mydriasis.
B Adrenaline-induced ocular hypotension is initially enhanced when used in combination with topical β-blockers.
C Topical cocaine causes anaesthesia, mydriasis and conjunctival blanching.
D Timolol applied topically to one eye also reduces the intraocular pressure of the unmedicated eye.
E Combined maintenance therapy of adrenaline and timolol has a strong ocular hypotensive effect.

7 Which of the following are correct?

A Combined oral β-blocker therapy is contraindicated with topical timolol.
B Thymoxamine is a competitive α-blocker.
C Thymoxamine reduces intraocular pressure.
D Guanethidine potentiates the effects of adrenaline in reducing intraocular pressure.
E Guanethidine reduces lid retraction found in thyroid eye disease.

8 Which of the following are true?

A Thymoxamine is of diagnostic value in angle closure glaucoma.
B Acetylcholine is available as a topical preparation and is effective in causing a complete miosis.
C Pilocarpine is a direct-acting ocular cholinergic agonist with no systemic side-effects.
D Pilocarpine reduces intraocular pressure mainly by increasing aqueous outflow.
E Pilocarpine should be given twice daily for control of intraocular pressure.

9 Carbachol

    A has a direct cholinergic action only
    B is a muscarinic and nicotinic agonist
    C is rapidly hydrolysed by cholinesterases
    D applied topically is an effective ocular hypotensive agent due to its high lipid solubility
    E causes vasodilatation

10 Which of the following statements about pilocarpine and physostigmine are true?

    A Brown eyes have a greater ocular hypotensive response to pilocarpine than blue eyes.
    B Ocular side-effects of pilocarpine include accommodative spasm, myopia and follicular conjunctivitis.
    C Physostigmine acts both centrally and peripherally as an irreversible cholinesterase inhibitor.
    D Physostigmine is both a muscarinic and nicotinic agonist.
    E Physostigmine solution undergoes a colour change due to oxidation when in storage.

11 Which of the following are true?

    A Physostigmine causes a ptosis, miosis and accommodative spasm.
    B Neostigmine is useful in treatment for *Phthirus pubis* infestation.
    C Physostigmine causes brow ache.
    D Edrophonium stimulates muscarinic receptors more than nicotinic receptors.
    E Edrophonium reduces intraocular pressure.

12 Which of the following are true?

    A Ecothiopate is a useful diagnostic and therapeutic tool in accommodative esotropia.
    B Low levels of plasma and red cell cholinesterase are always found in patients with systemic side-effects of cholinesterase inhibitors.
    C Systemic absorption of topically applied ocular drugs occurs mainly through ciliary vessels and Schlemm's canal.
    D Cyclopentolate causes mydriasis that lasts for 48 h.
    E Hyoscine causes mydriasis that lasts up to one week.

13 How many of the following statements about ecothiopate and atropine are true?

A Ecothiopate produces miosis that lasts for up to 4 weeks.
B Ecothiopate reduces intraocular pressure mainly by reducing aqueous production.
C Ecothiopate is associated with anterior subcapsular cataract.
D Atropine mydriasis lasts up to 48 h.
E Atropine is contraindicated in anterior uveitis.

14 Which of the following are true?

A Atropine-induced maximal mydriasis precedes cycloplegia.
B Homatropine causes mydriasis that is maximal in 40 min.
C Tropicamide causes mydriasis that recovers in 6 h.
D The degree of mydriasis due to tropicamide is independent of iris pigmentation.
E Atropine is also an α-adrenergic agonist.

15 Local anaesthetics

A are biphasic weak bases
B act on the cell membrane by maintaining a high permeability to sodium ions
C exhibit antimicrobial properties
D administered topically commonly cause desquamation of the corneal epithelium
E exhibit marked crossed hypersensitivity between different classes of anaesthetic

16 Glucocorticoids

A reduce numbers of neutrophils
B increase numbers of basophils
C reduce numbers of circulating red blood cells
D reduce numbers of eosinophils
E reduce numbers of monocytes

17 Which of these statements about steroids are true?

A Systemic corticosteroids reduce IgG and IgE titres.
B Steroids reduce numbers of B lymphocytes more than they reduce numbers of T lymphocytes.
C Glucocorticoids enter the cell membrane by receptor mediator transport.
D Plasma cortisol levels are lowest between 6 and 8 am.
E Topical ocular corticosteroids cause increased corneal thickness.

18 Ocular effects of corticosteroids include

    A increased intraocular pressure
    B posterior subcapsular cataract
    C neovascularization
    D miosis
    E ptosis

19 Which of the following statements about β-blockers are true?

    A Atenolol is a β_1-selective antagonist.
    B Betaxolol is a β_1-selective antagonist.
    C Levobunolol is a non-selective β-antagonist.
    D Propanolol is a β_1-selective antagonist.
    E Timolol is a non-selective β-antagonist.

20 Which of the following are true?

    A Topical propanolol causes corneal anaesthesia.
    B Timolol is available orally for the treatment of ocular hypertension.
    C Timolol has an additive ocular hypotensive effect when combined with pilocarpine.
    D Acetazolamide produces a metabolic alkalosis.
    E Topical acetazolamide penetrates the corneal epithelium poorly.

21 Acetazolamide

    A administered intravenously has a maximal ocular hypotensive effect within 5 min
    B 50% is found bound to plasma proteins
    C when protein bound is responsible for carbonic anhydrase inhibition
    D is metabolized in the liver
    E produces acidic urine

22 Acetazolamide

    A is a sulphonamide derivative
    B in combined therapy increases serum levels of phenytoin
    C is a useful adjunct in the treatment of petit mal epilepsy
    D is detected in the milk of lactating women being treated with acetazolamide
    E therapy causes depression

23 Acetazolamide

  A produces a metallic taste
  B therapy is associated with perioral paraesthesia
  C is associated with hypermetropia
  D is associated with urinary calculi
  E is associated with thrombocytopenia
  F is safe in patients with liver cirrhosis
  G is safe in pregnancy

24 Which of the following statements are true?

  A Urea exerts its hyperosmotic effect by remaining in the extracellular space.
  B Urea is metabolized by the kidney.
  C Oral mannitol is metabolized by the 'first-pass' phenomenon.
  D Seventy-five per cent of mannitol is protein bound in the extracellular space.
  E Glycerol has good penetration of the blood–aqueous barrier.
  F Glycerol exerts its hyperosmotic effect by inducing glycosuria.
  G Glycerol is well absorbed from the gastrointestinal tract.

25 Antibacterials: Penicillins

  A have a bactericidal effect
  B inhibit bacterial transpeptidases responsible for cross-linking polysaccharide chains
  C and cephalosporins contain a β-lactamase ring
  D cross the normal blood–ocular barrier easily
  E allergy is linked to cephalosporins, with 20% of people allergic to penicillin having cross-reactivity to cephalosporins

26 Antibacterials: Which of the following statements about cephalosporins are true?

  A β-Lactamase-producing *Staphylococcus aureus* is resistant to cephalosporins.
  B Third-generation cephalosporins have good penetration of the blood–brain barrier.
  C Third-generation cephalosporins have greater activity against β-lactamase gram-negative bacteria.
  D Cephadrine and cefadroxil are second-generation cephalosporins.
  E Cephalosporins are bacteriostatic.

27 Antibacterials: Which of the following statements about aminoglycosides are true?

    A Gentamicin acts by binding to bacterial ribosomes and inhibiting tRNA attachment.
    B Gentamicin easily crosses the normal blood–brain barrier.
    C Aminoglycosides are bactericidal.
    D Gentamicin ototoxicity destroys cochlear cells only.
    E Neomycin shows good absorption when administered orally.

28 Antibacterials: How many of these statements about tetracyclines are true?

    A Tetracycline binds to bacterial ribosomes and prevents tRNA and mRNA attachment.
    B Tetracycline is useful for the treatment of mycoplasma, Q fever and *Chlamydia*.
    C Tetracycline is effective in the treatment of 'corneal melting'.
    D Doxycycline is the only tetracycline excreted renally.
    E Oral tetracycline is the drug of choice in chlamydial ophthalmia neonatorum.
    F Tetracycline can potentiate Warfarin in combination therapy.

29 Erythromycin

    A is bacteriostatic
    B is effective in the treatment of *Mycoplasma pneumoniae*
    C easily crosses the blood–brain barrier and blood–ocular barriers
    D is associated with cholestatic jaundice
    E administered orally is the drug of choice for chlamydial ophthalmia neonatorum

30 Chloramphenicol

    A easily penetrates the blood–brain and blood–aqueous barrier
    B administered topically does not cause aplastic anaemia
    C is effective in the treatment of typhoid fever
    D is useful in the treatment of pneumonia
    E is effective in the treatment of CNS infections due to *Bacteroides fragilis*
    F is bacteriostatic

31 Metronidazole

    A acts by inhibiting RNA synthesis
    B may be administered by suppository to achieve satisfactory blood levels
    C is the treatment of choice for *Trichomonas vaginalis*
    D may be prescribed in pregnancy

E is useful in the treatment of anaerobic bacterial infections

F crosses the blood–brain barrier poorly

32 Which of the following statements about antifungal drugs are true?

A Nystatin is absorbed well through mucous membranes.

B Fluconazole is the drug of choice for CNS infections due to *Cryptococcus neoformans*.

C Flucytosine is usually used in combination with amphotericin B.

D Miconazole can be administered topically, subconjunctivally, orally and parenterally.

E Ketoconazole is known to be toxic to the eye when administered orally.

33 Antifungal drugs: Amphotericin B

A acts by altering the selective permeability of fungal cell membranes

B therapy is usually for 3–4 weeks

C cannot be administered topically

D intravenous administration is usually associated with unpleasant side-effects

E causes hypokalaemia

34 Antiviral drugs: Idoxuridine

A is useful in topical treatment of corneal dendritic ulcers

B treatment must be for at least 3 weeks

C reduces the risk of recurrence of herpesvirus

D is effective in the treatment of herpetic stromal keratitis

E applied systemically is highly toxic

35 Antiviral drugs: Acyclovir

A inhibits RNA polymerase in viral-infected cells

B is effective on its own against herpes simplex stromal keratitis

C administered orally is effective in the treatment of herpes zoster ophthalmicus

D administered intravenously commonly causes phlebitis at the injection site

E applied topically is effective in the treatment of genital herpes

36 Which of the following antibiotics are bactericidal?

A rifampicin
B chloramphenicol
C tetracycline
D ciprofloxacin
E trimethoprim
F sulphonamide
G co-trimoxazole

PHARMACOLOGY
Answers

1 **A** = True   **B** = True   **C** = True   **D** = True   **E** = True

Extraocular muscle palsy, pupillary abnormalities and ptosis occur after retrobulbar injection of local anaesthetic. Impairment of visual acuity is almost always found transiently. Conjunctival haemorrhage is common. Periocular administration of cortiosteroid has been reported to cause glaucoma, cataract, proptosis, Cushing's syndrome, systemic hypertension and retinal and choroidal vessel occlusion.

2 **A** = True   **B** = True   **C** = True   **D** = True   **E** = True

The corneal epithelium contains approximately two-thirds of the plasma membrane mass of the cornea. It therefore acts as a large store for lipophilic drugs whose release rate into the aqueous depends on their speed in altering to a hydrophilic phase.

The two main phases of detoxification and removal of drugs from the eye occur at the ciliary body. Phase 1 comprises the cytochrome p450 system that produces oxidation–reduction products. These are conjugated in phase 2. Melanin granules of the ciliary epithelium also provide a role in drug and toxin binding. Topical neomycin ointment can cause hypersensitivity reactions including blepharoconjunctivitis.

Topical drugs may have systemic side-effects due to their absorption into the bloodstream. Systemic side-effects of β-blockers include bronchospasm, bradycardia and systemic hypotension.

Subconjunctival injections are usually performed by passing a needle through the skin of the lid or through the inferior fornix. It is most useful in treatment of bacterial infection and severe uveitis, allowing high concentrations of antibiotics or steroids respectively.

3 **A** = True   **B** = True   **C** = True   **D** = True   **E** = True

Systemic digoxin therapy commonly causes colour vision disturbances. Although usually occurring within two weeks, they can occur as soon as day 1. The mechanism may be at a retinal level involving inhibition of the Na$^+$K$^+$ ATPase pump. This would also explain the impairment of dark adaptation and alteration in colour vision. Digoxin therapy has been shown to reduce intraocular pressure by 14% in patients with glaucoma. Aqueous formation has been shown to be reduced by 45%.

4 **A** = True   **B** = False   **C** = True   **D** = True   **E** = True

Noradrenaline is a water-soluble compound. Due to its polar nature the prior use of local anaesthetic is needed to increase the permeability of the lipid corneal epithelial barrier and allow greater penetration. Noradrenaline is a very effective ocular hypotensive agent and its main effect is on the aqueous outflow, perhaps by acting on the trabecular meshwork. It has very little effect on aqueous humour production. Phenylephrine is a synthetic amine similar to adrenaline, and is an α-agonist with no effect of note on β-receptors.

Timolol has a 24 h duration of action but is administered 12 hourly to avoid diurnal pressure variations.

5 **A** = False   **B** = True   **C** = True   **D** = True   **E** = False

Topical adrenaline causes conjunctival blanching, reduction in intraocular pressure and mydriasis without cycloplegia and so does not greatly alter visual acuity or reduce refractive changes. Due to the incidence of cystoid macular oedema, the use of adrenaline is contraindicated in aphakic eyes. It should also be avoided in subjects with narrow angles, cardiovascular disease, hyperthyroidism and subjects treated with monoamine oxidase inhibitors (MAOIs) or tricyclic antidepressants due to the increased sensitivity of adrenergic receptors.

Rebound miosis 24 h after installation of phenylephrine is often seen in patients over 50 years of age.

Hydroxyamphetamine is thought to release noradrenaline from adrenergic nerve terminals. Guanethidine depletes nerve terminals of noradrenaline and blocks the adrenergic effect of hydroxyamphetamine.

Pilocarpine and adrenaline are less effective in black subjects than white subjects in reducing intraocular pressure.

6 **A** = False   **B** = True   **C** = True   **D** = True   **E** = False

Low concentrations (1%) of adrenaline in the normal eye cause a triple response of conjunctival blanching, reduction of intraocular pressure and only slight mydriasis. The effects can be partly explained by its mixed α and β actions and poor corneal penetration. Combined therapy of adrenaline and timolol has an initial strong ocular hypotensive effect for about two weeks. With maintenance treatment beyond this period, this combined effect is lost. Combined maintenance therapy of timolol with either pilocarpine, dorzolamide, carbachol or acetazolamide, however, has a strong ocular hypotensive effect. One explanation is that timolol reduces aqueous production and eventually actually blocks the effect of adrenaline on outflow facility. Adrenaline is thought to increase outflow by β-receptor stimulation.

Aqueous flow can be thought of as an inflow and outflow. Both α- and β-receptors affect inflow and mainly β-receptors affect outflow. α-Receptor stimulation causes vasoconstriction of ciliary vasculature, reducing hydrostatic pressure and so reducing aqueous production (inflow). Stimulation of β-receptors increases aqueous production (inflow) by increasing cAMP in the non-pigmented ciliary epithelium. Stimulation of β-receptors in the outflow tracks increases outflow facility; stimulation of α-receptors has very little effect on outflow. β-blockade reduces inflow but has very little effect on outflow.

Cocaine acts as an anaesthetic by blocking conduction of nerve impulses. It has an adrenergic effect by blocking noradrenaline reuptake and so causes vasoconstriction and mydriasis. Systemically, it causes tachycardia, vasoconstriction and is a well-known CNS stimulant.

7 **A** = False   **B** = True   **C** = False   **D** = True   **E** = True

Combined therapy with oral β-blockers is not a contraindication to topical timolol as patients who tolerate β-blockers do not have problems with additional doses of topical timolol.

Thymoxamine produces miosis without any effect on the ciliary body and accommodation.

Guanethidine interferes with noradrenaline release from postganglionic adrenergic nerve endings. Its complex action is seen to initially cause noradrenaline release from nerve terminals soon followed by inhibition of both release and uptake. A curious hypersensitivity to adrenergic agonists is seen and thereby potentiation of their effects. Guanethidine is useful in the treatment of glaucoma due to its ability to reduce intraocular pressure for up to a month by both increasing outflow and reducing aqueous production.

When used in combination with adrenaline it has an enhancing effect of reducing intraocular pressure. Guanethidine is also useful in the treatment of Graves' disease-associated lid retraction.

8 **A** = True   **B** = False   **C** = False   **D** = True   **E** = False

Due to the fact that thymoxamine causes miosis without affecting intraocular pressure, aqueous outflow or aqueous production, it is useful in the diagnosis of acute closed-angle glaucoma. If by opening the angle of the anterior chamber by miosis, thymoxamine reduces intraocular pressure to normal, then the diagnosis of acute closed-angle glaucoma may be made. If intraocular pressure remains high or is only slightly reduced the diagnosis may be open-angle glaucoma or perhaps a combination of both. Acetylcholine is ineffective when applied topically it is available as a 1:100 preparation for use during surgical procedures and must be placed directly on the iris in order to achieve immediate and complete miosis of short duration.

Pilocarpine is an alkaloid of plant origin. It is a direct-acting muscarinic agonist with cholinergic effects on the cardiovascular system, central nervous system, exocrine glands and smooth muscle. It is thought to reduce intraocular pressure by contracting longitudinal muscles of the ciliary body affecting the scleral spur, widening the trabecular meshwork and so increasing aqueous outflow. Aqueous formation may also be slightly reduced with long-term use. Pilocarpine should be administered 3–4 times a day. Twice daily use of pilocarpine leads to inadequate control, especially if compounded by poor compliance.

9 **A** = False   **B** = True   **C** = False   **D** = False   **E** = True

Carbachol is resistant to hydrolysis by cholinesterases and so has a long direct-acting cholinergic effect. It also has indirect effect of displacing acetylcholine from nerve terminals. It stimulates both muscarinic and nicotinic receptors.

Carbachol is a very effective ocular hypotensive agent, but has poor lipid solubility and therefore requires the addition of 0.03% benzalkonium chloride (BAK) preservative to aid corneal penetration or 0.005% BAK along with 1% hydroxypropyl methylcellulose to prolong ocular surface contact.

Carbachol causes brief vasodilation and therefore short-lasting conjunctival and ciliary injection. To avoid the risk of increasing inflammation, it is therefore contraindicated in patients with anterior uveitis and neovascular glaucoma.

10 **A** = False   **B** = True   **C** = False   **D** = True   **E** = True

Brown pigmented eyes show a reduced ocular hypotensive response to pilocarpine than blue eyes due to pigment binding. These patients often require higher concentration solutions. Although the hypotensive effect is reduced in pigmented eyes, the subsequent release of pilocarpine from the pigment provides a more prolonged response.

Physostigmine is a highly lipid-soluble reversible cholinesterase inhibitor that is easily able to cross the blood–brain barrier and so exert both a peripheral and central effect on both muscarinic and nicotinic receptors.

Aqueous solutions of physostigmine are usually stored after sterilization with antioxidants at a buffered pH of less than 4. Oxidation is seen to turn the colourless solution pink and reduce efficacy.

11 **A** = False   **B** = False   **C** = True   **D** = False   **E** = False

Physostigmine causes miosis that begins after 5 min, is maximal at 30 min and lasts for 4 h. It also causes accommodative spasm that begins after 20 min and lasts for 3 h. It also causes conjunctival vasodilation and a reduction in intraocular pressure. It does not produce ptosis. Physostigmine has antimicrobial properties related to its anticholinesterase action against *Phthirus pubis*. Side-effects of physostigmine include lid twitching (nicotinic receptors), accommodative spasm, myopia, brow ache and allergic follicular conjunctivitis.

Edrophonium (Tensilon) is a reversible cholinesterase inhibitor. It predominantly stimulates nicotinic receptors and acts on the neuromuscular junction. Ideal for the diagnosis of myasthenia gravis, it transiently increases muscle strength when administered intravenously (Tensilon Test). Tonography has shown that edrophonium causes a brief rise in intraocular pressure of up to 5 mmHg.

12 A = True **B** = True **C** = False **D** = False **E** = True

Ecothiophate is an irreversible cholinesterase inhibitor. By potentiating acetylcholine it allows less effort in accommodation and so less accommodative convergence. In patients with esotropia, an accommodative component can be implicated if the patient corrects his or her visual axis with ecothiopate. Continuing on a lower dose for up to 2 years can be an effective treatment.

Systemic absorption of cholinesterase inhibitors results in low levels of plasma and red cell cholinesterase levels. Normal levels rule out drug-related symptoms.

Systemic absorption of topically applied ocular drugs occurs mainly through conjunctival vessels and the nasal mucosa. It is therefore useful to manually compress the lacrimal canaliculi after installation of a drug in order to reduce systemic side-effects.

Cyclopentolate is a water-soluble anticholinergic drug. One per cent cyclopentolate causes maximum mydriasis in 30 min and maximum cycloplegia within 60 min. Residual accommodation is approximately 1.25 dioptres. Mydriasis and cycloplegia return to normal within 24 h.

Hyoscine (scopolamine) is a potent anticholinergic drug with similar efficacy to atropine. Maximum mydriasis occurs in 20 min. Maximum cycloplegia occurs in 40 min (residual accommodation being 1.6 dioptres) and returns to normal in 3 days. Mydriasis returns to normal in 7 days.

13 A = True **B** = False **C** = True **D** = False **E** = False

Ecothiopate is an irreversible cholinesterase inhibitor with poor lipid solubility. Topical ecothiophate causes miosis from 10 to 45 min lasting up to four weeks.

Ecothiopate reduces intraocular pressure for up to 4 days, mainly by increasing aqueous outflow facility. More than other cholinesterases, it is associated with the onset of cataract. Anterior subcapsular cataracts are commonly associated but nuclear sclerotic and posterior subcapsular cataract may also be accelerated. Atropine, first isolated from the plant *Atropa belladonna* is a naturally occurring alkaloid. It is one of the most potent cholinergic antagonists available and causes strong mydriasis maximal at 30 min and lasting up to 10 days. It causes cycloplegia that is maximal in 3 h and lasts for 7 days.

Atropine relaxes ciliary muscle spasm reducing pain, it prevents posterior synechiae by maximally dilating the pupil and reducing convexity and thickness of the lens, and it also plays a role in reducing the vasodilation and permeability of inflamed leaking vessels. It is therefore useful in the treatment of anterior uveitis.

14 **A** = True **B** = True **C** = True **D** = True **E** = True

Homatropine is an anticholinergic drug of one-tenth potency of atropine. It causes maximum mydriasis and weaker cycloplegia in 40 min. Recovery is complete within 3 days.

Tropicamide is a predominantly unionized anticholinergic drug. Its resultant lipid solubility explains its fast action. One per cent tropicamide produces maximal mydriasis in 20 min and maximal cycloplegia in 30 min. Full recovery is within 6 h. Tropicamide-induced mydriasis appears to be independent of iris pigmentation or racial differences.

Atropine is thought to cause mydriasis both by blocking muscarinic receptors on the sphincter pupillae muscle and mildly stimulating α-adrenergic receptors on the dilator pupillae muscle.

15 **A** = True **B** = False **C** = True **D** = True **E** = False

Local anaesthetics are locally applied reversible drugs that block nerve conduction resulting in loss of sensation. Structurally, they consist of an aromatic lipophilic portion linked to an intermediate aliphatic chain by an ester or amide linkage. This is followed by a nitrogen-containing hydrophilic hydrocarbon chain. They are weak bases with a pK_a between 8 and 9.

In solution they are ionized and water soluble, but at a neutral pH they become unionized and penetrate tissue.

Local anaesthetics block nerve conduction by acting on the cell membrane and blocking the rise in permeability to sodium ions, thereby preventing sodium influx across the membrane. Local anaesthetics have been shown to exhibit antimicrobial properties. Tetracaine inhibits the growth of *Staphylococcus aureus*, *Candida albicans* and *Pseudomonas*.

Local anaesthetics applied topically to the eye can cause localized or diffuse corneal epithelial desquamation within 5 min.

16 **A** = False **B** = False **C** = False **D** = True **E** = True

Glucocorticorticoids cause neutrophilia, but neutrophil migration is inhibited.

17 **A** = False **B** = False **C** = False **D** = False **E** = True

IgE may be considered a mediator of the allergic response and IgG may be considered a mediator of the autoimmune response. Systemic corticosteroids do not affect IgG or IgE titres. Glucocorticoids reduce allergic type 1 hypersensitivity by reducing histamine and prostaglandin production. Corticosteroids reduce numbers of lymphocytes with a greater in reduction T lymphocytes than in B lymphocytes.

Glucocorticoids pass through cell membranes without the need for receptor-mediated transport. They bind to intracellular receptors and signal the nucleus to either upregulate or downregulate protein synthesis.

Plasma cortisol levels are highest between 6 and 8 am. They are lowest around midnight.

18 **A** = True   **B** = True   **C** = False   **D** = False   **E** = True

Ocular effects of corticosteroids include corneal thickening and vasoconstriction of conjunctival vessels and the inhibition of both corneal epithelial healing and neovascularization.

Protein and glucose levels in aqueous and vitreous compartments are elevated with urea and ascorbic acid levels reduced. Intraocular pressure is raised with a greater rise in patients with glaucoma than normal subjects.

Corticosteroids are cataractogenic and are associated with an increased incidence of posterior subcapsular cataract. An increase in lens hydration is seen with increased lens sodium levels and reduced potassium, urea and glutathione levels.

Topical corticosteroids are associated with mild mydriasis (1 mm) and mild ptosis. Brief ocular discomfort is a common complaint with topical steroids. They have also been shown to occasionally cause refractive errors.

Superimposed infection by bacteria, fungi and viruses is a recognized and obvious risk, and if present contraindicates the use of corticosteroids.

The benefits of corticosteroids are evident in ocular inflammation where they have a non-specific anti-inflammatory effect in reducing capillary permeability and exudate. They inhibit neutrophil migration, fibroblast growth and toxic enzyme release to dampen inflammation.

19 **A** = True   **B** = True   **C** = True   **D** = False   **E** = True

Atenolol is a selective β_1-antagonist administered orally as a 50 mg daily tablet for the treatment of systemic hypertension. It has been shown to reduce intraocular pressure by 35% approximately 5 h after ingestion for about 7 h. Betaxolol (Betoptic) is a β_1-selective antagonist available as ophthalmic drops for topical use only. It produces a 30% reduction in intraocular pressure within 2 h and this lasts for up to 12 h. Its selectivity reduces the risk of systemic side-effects of β_2-blockade (bronchoconstriction and exacerbation of chronic obstructive airways disease (COAD)).

Levobunalol (Betagan) is a non-selective β-antagonist available as an ophthalmic solution for topical use only. It has a long duration of action with 26–30% maximal reduction of intraocular pressure lasting up to 24 h. It is administered twice daily.

Propanolol is a non-selective β-antagonist available for oral and intravenous use in the treatment of systemic hypertension, angina, certain cardiac arrhythmias, hypertrophic cardiomyopathies and migraine headaches. It produces a dose-dependent reduction in intraocular pressures.

Timolol (Timoptol) is a non-selective β-antagonist. Due to the predominance of β_2-receptors in the eye a β_2-antagonist effect is seen.

20 **A** = True **B** = False **C** = True **D** = False **E** = True

Propranolol has strong membrane-stabilizing properties and so acts as a local anaesthetic. Topical application of propranolol causes significant corneal anaesthesia.

Oral timolol has a dose-related ocular hypotensive effect. It is available for the treatment of systemic hypertension with patients on oral timolol; further reduction in intraocular pressure is not achieved with combined topical timolol. Miotics such as pilocarpine have an additive ocular hypotensive effect when combined with timolol. Both may be administered twice daily.

Acetazolamide is a carbonic anhydrase inhibitor. It reduces intraocular pressure by inhibiting the production of bicarbonate, and reducing the amount of sodium and chloride entering into the posterior chamber. This has the effect of reducing aqueous humour production. By inhibiting bicarbonate production, acetazolamide has an effect on renal function and acid-base equilibrium of a mild metabolic acidosis. Topical acetazolamide has poor corneal penetration and only produces a very small reduction in intraocular pressure. Dorzolamide has been recently introduced as a topical carbonic anhydrase inhibitor.

21 **A** = False **B** = False **C** = False **D** = False **E** = False

Acetazolamide is available in both oral and intravenous forms. Orally, its onset of action is in 1 h, maximally reducing intraocular pressure between 2 and 4 h, and lasting for up to 6 h. Intravenously, its onset of action is in 1 min with a maximum reduction within 30 min lasting for up to 4 h. A sustained-release twice daily oral capsule is also available, which maximally reduces intraocular pressure for up to 12 h and lasts up to 18 h. Up to 95% of acetazolamide in the circulation is plasma protein bound. Fifty per cent of unbound acetazolamide is unionized and is responsible for cell penetration and carbonic anhydrase inhibition.

Acetazolamide is not metabolized. It is excreted renally by the proximal convoluted tubule into urine.

22 **A** = True **B** = True **C** = True **D** = True **E** = True

Acetazolamide is a sulphonamide derivative and is contraindicated in patients with sulphonamide hypersensitivity. Combined therapy with phenytoin results in modification of phenytoin metabolism and increased phenytoin serum levels. One of the indications of acetazolamide therapy is adjunct in the treatment of petit mal epilepsy.

Acetazolamide is detected in the milk of lactating women being treated with acetazolamide and so is not recommended during breastfeeding. A recognized side-effect with acetazolamide therapy is mild depression.

23 **A** = True   **B** = True   **C** = False   **D** = True   **E** = True   **F** = False   **G** = False

Acetazolamide has both ocular and systemic side-effects. Ocular side-effects include myopia, probably due to shallowing of the anterior chamber secondary to forward shift of the lens and iris and caused by ciliary body oedema. Systemic side-effects include peripheral and perioral paresthesia, metallic taste, malaise, loss of libido, abdominal cramps and metabolic acidosis.

Acetazolamide causes increased urinary bicarbonate levels and decreased urinary citrate level, producing alkaline urine. This increases the risk of calcium phosphate urinary calculi. Alkalinization of urine reduces excretion of ammonium (NH_4^+). Increased blood ammonia levels carry a risk of hepatic encephalopathy in patients with liver failure.

Although acetazolamide has not been implicated in human congenital defects, it is teratogenic in animals and so is not recommended in pregnancy.

24 **A** = False   **B** = False   **C** = False   **D** = False   **E** = False   **F** = False   **G** = True

Due to its solubility, urea is distributed all over the body, including the eye. It is found in both intra- and extracellular spaces and both intra- and extravascular spaces. It is excreted by the kidney and urine. Mannitol is a hyperosmolar agent that remains unbound to protein in the extracelluar fluid compartment and produces diuresis and cellular dehydration. It is excreted 90% unchanged by the kidney in urine. Oral mannitol is not absorbed by the gastrointestinal tract.

Glycerol is an orally administered hyperosmotic agent. It penetrates poorly the unin-flamed blood–aqueous barrier. It has a calorific value and can cause hyperglycaemia in patients with diabetes. Hyperosmotic agents are effective in reducing intraocular pressure. They cause a rapid rise in plasma osmolality, thereby resulting in a fluid shift from the vitreous and aqueous into the plasma.

25 **A** = True   **B** = True   **C** = False   **D** = False   **E** = False

Penicillins are bactericidal by inhibiting bacterial cell wall synthesis. Along with cephalosporins they are β-lactam-containing antibiotics and have variable susceptibility to β-lactamases produced by certain bacteria.

Penicillins along with first- and second-generation cephalosporins do not easily cross the normal blood–brain or blood–ocular barriers. They do, however, cross the inflamed blood–brain barrier easily. They are actively transported out of the aqueous by the ciliary body.

Ten per cent of people allergic to penicillin have cross-reactivity to cephalosporins.

26 **A** = False **B** = True **C** = True **D** = False **E** = False

Cephalosporins are bactericidal antibiotics that interfere with cell wall synthesis by preventing cross-linking in a similar way to penicillin. They also contain a β-lactam ring. Cephalosporins are usually active against β-lactamase (penicillinase)-producing *Staphylococcus aureus* and are inactivated by gram-negative bacteria producing β-lactamase. First-generation cephalosporins include cephradine, cephalexin and cefadroxil. They have good gram-positive cover and not so good activity against gram-negative bacteria. They are easily inactivated by gram-negative bacteria producing β-lactamase and cross the blood–brain barrier poorly.

Second-generation cephalosporins include cefuroxime, cefaclor and cefoxitin. They have greater gram-negative activity and are useful in treating infections due to gram-positive cocci, *Haemophilus influenzae*, *Enterobacter*, *Proteus*, *E. coli* and *Klebsiella*. They have some activity against anaerobes such as *Bacteroides*.

Unlike first- and second-generation cephalosporins, third-generation cephalosporins such as cefotaxime, ceftriaxone, and ceftazidime have good blood–brain and blood–ocular barrier penetration. Third-generation cephalosporins have reduced activity against gram-positive bacteria, but have increased resistance to β-lactamase produced by gram-negative bacteria. They are extremely useful in treating gram-negative infections due to *Pseudomonas*, *E. coli*, *Klebsiella*, *Proteus*, *Haemophilus influenzae*, *Enterobacter* and *Serratia*, which include gram-negative bacillary meningitis, abdominal or pelvic infections, lower respiratory tract infections and septicaemia.

27 **A** = True **B** = False **C** = True **D** = False **E** = False

Aminoglycosides such as gentamicin prevent protein synthesis by binding to bacterial ribosomes and inhibiting tRNA and mRNA binding as well as causing codon-misreading. Gentamicin is useful for treatment of gram-negative bacillary infections. It crosses the inflamed blood–brain barrier and is useful in the treatment of meningitis. Due to its water solubility it crosses the normal blood–brain barrier poorly and does not penetrate the normal cornea well. It is therefore extremely useful in the treatment of external bacterial eye disease and bacterial corneal ulcers. Gentamicin ototoxicity affects both cochlea cells (tinnitus, pressure sensation) and vestibular cells (nystagmus, vertigo, nausea, vomiting).

Nephrotoxicity in the form of acute tubular necrosis occurs with very high concentrations.

Neomycin is one of the most toxic aminoglycosides. It has very few indications for intravenous administration. Due to its poor gut absorption, oral administration is useful in bowel preparation for surgery or in the treatment of hepatic encephalopathy. It is commonly administered topically for external ear and skin bacterial infections.

28 **A** = True   **B** = True   **C** = True   **D** = False   **E** = False   **F** = True

Tetracycline inhibits protein synthesis in human and bacterial cells by ribosomal bind-ing. It is not taken up actively in human cells.

Tetracyclines have a broad spectrum of action against gram-positive, gram-negative and both aerobic and anaerobic bacteria. They are useful in the treatment of *Myco-plasma pneumoniae* infection, rickettsial infections (typhus and Q fever) and chlamydial infections (*C. trachomatis*).

Tetracycline has an effective role in the treatment of sterile non-infected corneal ulcers ('corneal melting') in which stromal necrosis is thought to be due to collagenase activity. Tetracycline is thought to have anticollagenase properties.

Doxycycline is the only tetracycline excreted mainly by the gastrointestinal tract. The majority of tetracyclines are excreted renally and are contraindicated in renal impairment.

Tetracyclines may be used topically in the treatment of chlamydial ophthalmia neo-natorum but systemic erythromycin is the drug of choice. In children below the age of 8 years tetracycline slows bone growth and causes changes in dentition including dis-coloration and dysgenesis due to the formation of tetracycline–calcium phosphate complexes.

29 **A** = False   **B** = True   **C** = False   **D** = True   **E** = True

Erythromycin is a bactericidal antibiotic. It is effective in the treatment of atypical pneumonias such as that caused by *Mycoplasma pneumoniae*, *Coxiella burnetii*, *Legionella pneumophila*, or as an alternative to penicillin in streptococcal infections.

Erythromycin crosses the blood–brain and blood–ocular barriers poorly. Cholestatic jaundice is a rare but recognized complication of erythromycin therapy.

30 **A** = True   **B** = False   **C** = True   **D** = True   **E** = True   **F** = True

Chloramphenicol is a bacteriostatic antibiotic containing the key toxic element nitro-benzene. It acts by competing with mRNA for binding on to bacterial ribosomes and inhibiting protein synthesis. It has a broad spectrum of gram-positive and gram-nega-tive activity and is effective against *Haemophilus influenzae*, *Neisseria*, *Yersinia pestis* (plague) and anaerobes as well as having some action against *Streptococcus pneu-moniae*, staphylococci and most gram-negative bacilli (except *Pseudomonas*). Due to its high lipid solubility it penetrates the cornea, blood–aqueous barrier and blood–brain easily. It is therefore an effective topical antibiotic, and the drug of choice for CNS infections (including those due to *Bacteroides fragilis*).

Chloramphenicol is highly effective against most *Salmonella* infections, including typhoid fever. It may be used for the treatment of pneumonia due to *Haemophilus influenzae*, but due to its toxic side-effects it is not the drug of choice.

Chloramphenicol has a dose-related side-effect of reversible bone marrow depression causing anaemia, reduced erythrocyte iron uptake and raised serum iron levels. Patients taking systemic or topical chloramphenicol carry a very small risk of the more serious idiosyncratic side-effect of aplastic anaemia. This occurs months after completion and results in irreversible pancytopenia. It is worth noting that the topical dose of chloramphenicol is a fraction of the oral dose.

31 **A** = False **B** = True **C** = True **D** = False **E** = True **F** = False

Metronidazole is a nitroimidazole with a bactericidal action against anaerobic bacteria such as *Bacteroides*. It is also the drug of choice in the treatment of amoebiasis, *Trichomonas vaginalis* and giardiasis. It acts by inhibiting microbial DNA synthesis. Although metronidazole has not been proven to be teratogenic in humans, animal experiments have shown nitroimidazoles to be carcinogenic, and so the use is contra-indicated in pregnancy. It is recommended that alcohol be avoided whilst taking metronidazole due to the interaction with ethanol producing an unpleasant acetaldehyde intoxication and histamine release.

Metronidazole has excellent penetration of the blood–brain barrier.

32 **A** = False **B** = True **C** = True **D** = true **E** = False

Nystatin (<u>N</u>ew <u>Y</u>ork <u>STAT</u>e) is useful in the treatment of oral, enteric and vaginal candidiasis. Hypersensitivity, mucous membrane irritation, blood interactions or serious systemic side-effects have not been reported.

Fluconazole is an imidazole antifungal agent active against aerobic organisms. It penetrates the blood–brain barrier well and is useful in the treatment of infections due to *Cryptococcus neoformans*.

Flucytosine is a fluorinated pyrimidine derivative that is converted to fluorouracil in fungal cells and not in host cells. Useful in infections by *Cryptococcus neoformans* and *Candida* (including endophthalmitis), it is used in combination with amphotericin B due to the high incidence of resistance. It has good blood–brain barrier penetration but can be hepatotoxic as well as causing bone marrow suppression.

Miconazole is a broad-spectrum imidazole with a fungi static effect, especially in low doses, affecting permeability, as well as a fungicidal effect. It can be administered topically to skin for the treatment of dermatophytosis. It is effective in the treatment of corneal fungal infections when administered topically, subconjunctivally or systemically. It is active both orally and parentally. It is often used in combination with amphotericin B for severe systemic fungal infections.

Ketoconazole is an antifungal imidazole effective against chronic candidiasis and dermatophytosis when applied topically and when administered orally, in the treatment of deep systemic mycoses due to aspergillosis, cryptococcosis, histoplasmosis, candidiasis and blastomycosis. Side-effects include reversible liver damage that has been fatal in at least one case, and more commonly nausea and pruritus. Ketoconazole is not toxic to the eye when administered orally. It can cause irritation when applied topically in the treatment of corneal fungal infection.

33 **A** = True   **B** = False   **C** = False   **D** = True   **E** = True

Amphotericin B is a potent polyene antifungal agent that can be used intravenously in severe deep systemic fungal infections as well as in a dilute form for topical administration in fungal corneal ulcers. It acts by binding to sterols in the fungal cell membrane and altering the selective permeability of the membrane to facilitate the leaking out of intracellular solutes.

Amphotericin is ineffective against bacteria due to the absence of sterols in their cell membrane. Unfortunately, due to the presence of sterols in renal tubular cells and red blood cells, Amphotericin binding causes nephrotoxicity and reversible anaemia. Hypokalaemia and hypomagnasaemia may also be seen. Amphotericin is a very unpleasant drug when administered intravenously, causing discomfort, nausea, pyrexia, rigors and headaches.

Treatment of systemic infections is usefully continued for 6–10 weeks but can be for as long as four months.

34 **A** = True   **B** = False   **C** = False   **D** = False   **E** = True

Idoxuridine is a thymidine analogue and is active against herpes simplex virus. It creates fraudulent DNA both in the host cells and the virus. It is useful in topical treatment of dendritic ulcers of the corneal epithelium. Seventy-five per cent of patients are cured within two weeks. Treatment should not be continued for more than three weeks due to toxicity. Idoxuridine does not reduce the risk of recurrence.

Due to water insolubility, Idoxuridine shows poor penetration of the corneal stroma. It is ineffective in the treatment of herpes stromal keratitis. Due to its high toxicity to host cells, systemic use is extremely limited. It is available as 0.1% topical eye solution, and a 5% solution with dimethyl sulphoxide (DMSO) for topical skin application, but these have generally been superseded by more recent preparations and are thought to be of little use.

35 **A** = False   **B** = False   **C** = True   **D** = True   **E** = True

Acyclovir is a guanosine analogue. This is activated only through phosphorylation by herpes thymidine kinase. The activated phosphate inhibits the DNA polymerase of herpes-infected cells. Thymidine kinase is induced in virally infected cells and remains stable in non-infected host cells. Acyclovir therefore remains inactive in the presence of non-infected cells.

Acyclovir is effective against herpes simplex virus and herpes zoster virus.

Although highly successful in the treatment of herpetic corneal dendritic ulcers, topical acyclovir on its own is not so effective in penetrating and treating stromal keratitis. Combined steroid therapy is indicated.

Acyclovir 800 mg five times a day for 7 days is an effective treatment for herpes zoster ophthalmicus, especially in conjunction with topical ointment.

Side-effects of acyclovir include mild burning, stinging or itching when applied topically, nausea, diarrhoea, headache and arthralgia when taken orally, and phlebitis and renal impairment with intravenous administration.

36 **A** = True   **B** = False   **C** = False   **D** = True   **E** = False   **F** = False   **G** = False

Rifampicin has a bactericidal action by binding to DNA-dependent RNA polymerase and inhibiting initiation of transcription.

Chloramphenicol has a bacteriostatic action inhibiting translation.

Tetracycline has a bacteriostatic action inhibiting translation.

Ciprofloxacin is quinolone that has a bactericidal action inhibiting the enzyme responsible for bacterial DNA coiling.

Trimethoprim has a bacteriostatic action by inhibiting bacterial dihydrofolate reductase and preventing new nucleic acid synthesis.

Sulphonamides have a bacteriostatic action by acting as analogues of para-aminobenzoic acid and inhibiting folic acid synthesis.

Co-trimoxazole is a combination of trimethoprim and the sulphonamide sulphamethoxazole. It incorporates the bacteriostatic actions of both trimethoprim and the sulphonamide.

PATHOLOGY
Questions

1 Acute increase in cell volume may be due to

A reduced phospholipids
B intracellular hypoxia
C inhibition of protein synthesis
D lack of ATP
E failure of cell surface ion pumps

2 Which of the following statements about cell injury are true?

A The commonest cell changes in non-lethal cell injury are increased cell volume and intracellular fat accumulation.
B There is loss of calcium ions from the cell in cell death.
C There is loss of phospholipid by the cell in ischaemic injury.
D Apoptosis describes degeneration of a cell in which metabolic activity is reduced but not abolished.
E Aseptic necrosis describes the death of bone due to ischaemia.

3 With regard to cell injury, which of the following are true?

A Nitrosamines cause cell injury by methylation of DNA and RNA.
B Cyanide causes cell injury by combining with iron of cytochrome oxidase.
C Methanol is toxigenic by its conversion to formaldehyde.
D Epidermal cells of xeroderma pigmentosa cannot repair damage due to X-rays.
E A free radical is a molecule with a single unpaired electron in its outer orbit.

4 Which of the following chemical mediators act as chemotactic factors?

A Leukotriene B_4
B Complement C5a
C Interleukin 1 (IL-I)
D Tumour necrosis factor (TNF)
E Interleukin 8 (IL-8)

5 Chemical mediators that cause increased vascular permeability include

    A platelet-activating factor
    B kinins
    C lysosomal cationic proteins
    D histamine
    E complement C3a and C5a
    F leukotriene B_4

6 Chemical mediators directly causing vasodilation include

    A prostaglandin I_2
    B kinins
    C interleukin 1
    D bacterial endotoxin
    E histamine
    F Nitric oxide

7 Effects of interleukin 1 include

    A osteoclast stimulation
    B stimulation of fibroblast proliferation and collagen synthesis
    C B and T cell activation
    D increased neutrophil production of interleukin 1
    E fever
    F increased synthesis of acute-phase proteins by hepatocytes
    G reduced albumin synthesis by hepatocytes

8 Phagocytosis is a function of

    A macrophages
    B eosinophils
    C basophils
    D plasma cells
    E neutrophils
    F mast cells

9 In acute inflammation, mast cells release

    A histamine
    B heparin

C platelet-activating factor
D tumour necrosis factor α (TNF-α)
E fibrin

10 Which of the following statements about inflammation are true?

A Denervation of local arterioles markedly reduces the acute inflammatory response.
B IgG and complement C3b are opsonins of neutrophils and macrophages.
C Interleukin 2 is produced by activated macrophages.
D Abscess formation implies progression to chronic inflammation.
E Increased vascular permeability within the first 30 min of inflammation occurs in venules only.

11 Which of the following statements about chronic inflammation are true?

A Increased plasma cells are seen in chronic inflammation.
B The lifespan of a tissue macrophage is 72 h.
C Granulomatous inflammation implies increased production of granulation tissue.
D A granuloma implies the presence of three or more macrophage-derived cells.
E Marked tissue destruction is a feature of chronic inflammation.
F Chronic inflammation is associated with amyloid deposition.

12 Interferon

A production is most strongly stimulated by single-stranded viral DNA
B γ is produced by virally infected leukocytes
C inhibits translation of viral mRNA
D is specific for an individual virus
E induces fever
F increases cell surface expression of both MHC (major histocompatibility complex) class I and class II antigens
G activates macrophages

13 With regard to complement, which of the following are true?

A The alternative pathway describes the formation of C1qrs complex.
B The classical pathway is antibody dependent.
C C3 is the most abundant component of the complement proteins.
D Two or more antibodies bound to a microbe are required to trigger the complement cascade.
E IgG, IgM or IgE are required to directly trigger the complement cascade.

14 Acute-phase proteins include

   A fibrinogen
   B C-reactive protein
   C serum amyloid A protein
   D factor VIII
   E ferritin

15 In type I hypersensitivity,

   A raised serum IgE levels are associated with atopy
   B late response is due to flare and weal
   C IL-4 induces IgE production by B lymphocytes
   D macrophages play no role in triggering IgE production
   E systemic anaphylaxis is due to massive activation of IgE-producing plasma cells

16 Type II hypersensitivity

   A is seen in Goodpasture's syndrome
   B is responsible for acute transplant rejection
   C involves activation of complement
   D is associated with a positive Coomb's test
   E requires IgM or IgG

17 Type III hypersensitivity

   A involves platelet aggregation
   B is a result of formation of soluble antigen/antibody complexes
   C is associated with glomerulonephritis
   D is characterized by polymorphonuclear leukocyte infiltration
   E results in complement-mediated tissue damage

18 Which of the following statements about type IV hypersensitivity are true?

   A Type IV hypersensitivity may be transferred by serum to non-sensitized subjects.
   B T cells express the CD3 receptor.
   C The major histocompatibility complex is a gene locus found on chromosome 8.
   D Class II human leukocyte antigens are found on macrophages and B cells.
   E CD8 cells recognize antigens associated with class I MHC molecules.

19 With regard to transplant immunology,

   A corneal grafting usually involves transplant of an isograft
   B acute rejection is a cell-mediated immune response
   C cyclosporin A acts mainly by inhibiting antigen-activated CD8 cells
   D acute rejection is mediated by passenger leukocytes acting as class I major histocompatibility antigens
   E hyperacute rejection occurs mainly in association with xenograft donor tissue

20 Atherosclerosis

   A describes atheromatous plaque deposition on to the endothelium
   B involves smooth muscle cell proliferation in the intima
   C may be complicated by aneurysm due to thinning of the underlying media
   D may be complicated by plaque ulceration
   E is associated with raised levels of HDL (high-density lipoprotein)

21 Thrombosis is associated with

   A laminar blood flow
   B homocystinuria
   C cardiac failure
   D sickle cell anaemia
   E protein C deficiency
   F temporal arteritis
   G polyarteritis nodosa
   F stasis

22 Infarction

   A histologically is usually wedge-shaped
   B in the first hour shows a darker colour than normal
   C except in the brain is followed by coagulative necrosis
   D is associated with venous occlusion
   F may precede abscess formation

23 Which of the following statements about oedema are true?

   A Transudate contains predominantly fibrinogen with low levels of albumin.
   B Pulmonary oedema is associated with acute raised intracranial pressure.
   C Oedema may be seen in shock.

D Filariasis causes oedema of the external genitalia and lower limbs.

E Hypoalbuminaemia is associated with hyperaldosteronism.

24 With regard to pigmentation,

A lipofuscins are found in the heart and liver

B bilirubin is seen binding to scleral proteins in jaundice

C haemosiderin accumulation is responsible for the dark blue colour of a bruise

D abnormal melanin metabolism is seen in alcaptonuria

E lipofuscin is toxic to cells

25 With regard to heterotrophic calcification, which of the following are true?

A Dystrophic calcification describes both intracellular and extracellular calcium deposition.

B Psammoma bodies are usually seen in association with metastatic calcification.

C Old cerebral haemorrhages are associated with calcification.

D Metastatic calcification occurs in normal tissue due to hypercalcaemia.

E Metastatic calcification is seen in atherosclerosis.

F Dystrophic calcification is seen in tuberculosis.

26 Which of the following statements about neoplasia are correct?

A Benign neoplasms contain a high number of cells undergoing mitosis.

B Nuclei in malignant neoplasia are hyperchromatic.

C Pleomorphism is a feature of malignant neoplasms.

D Malignant neoplasms always invade surrounding tissue.

E Benign neoplasms are well differentiated.

F Benign neoplasms may be fatal.

27 In neoplasia,

A dysplasia means irreversible reduction in cell differentiation without invasion

B carcinoma *in situ* is defined as epithelial dysplasia in all layers with early basement membrane invasion

C hamartoma is a non-neoplastic congenital malformation

D dysplasia describes tissue metaplasia

E a polyp is defined as a neoplastic pedunculated cell mass arising from an epithelial surface

28 In non-neoplastic proliferation,

    A the restriction point in the G_1 phase of the cell cycle refers to termination of DNA polymerase synthesis
    B the S phase of the cell cycle has a constant length
    C hyperplasia is usually under negative feedback control
    D hypertrophy refers to increase in size of cells only
    E hyperplasia is never pathological
    F hypertrophy may be due to cellular swelling or oedema

29 Tumour spread involves

    A reduced cell surface expression of laminin receptors
    B type IV collagenase activity
    C fibroblast growth factor (FGF) release
    D loss of anchorage dependence
    F increased fibronectin expression on cell surface

30 Which if the following statements about carcinogenesis are true?

    A The initiation step in carcinogenesis is irreversible.
    B Human papillomavirus types 6 and 11 predispose to carcinoma of the cervix.
    C Polycyclic aromatic hydrocarbons predispose to skin cancer.
    D Saccharine predisposes to bladder cancer.
    E UV-A is the most potent ultraviolet carcinogen.
    F Ionizing radiation exposure predisposes to thyroid carcinoma.

31 With regard to oncogenes,

    A proto-oncogenes are normal genes signalling DNA sequences
    B the *erb*B oncogene codes for a transmembrane growth factor receptor
    C the *ras* oncogene codes for the cell-signalling G protein
    D they may be activated by translocation of a proto-oncogene
    E they may be carried by viruses

32 With regard to tumour markers, which of the following associations are correct?

    A CA125 and ovarian tumours
    B AFP (α-fetoprotein) and hepatocellular carcinoma
    C CRP (C-reactive protein) and breast cancer
    D CEA (carcinoembryonic antigen) and colonic carcinoma

E amylase and pancreatic carcinoma
D acid phosphatase and prostatic carcinoma

33 Amyloid

A is a carbohydrate arranged in β-pleated sheets
B bound to Congo Red dye shows dichroism in polarized light
C structure is related to the Bence-Jones protein
D precursor is an acute-phase protein
E causes restrictive cardiomyopathy
F deposition in the brain is seen in all patients over 40 years of age with Down's syndrome
G deposition is associated with acute inflammation

PATHOLOGY
Answers

1 **A** = False   **B** = True   **C** = False   **D** = True   **E** = True

See notes on Pathology Question 2.

2 **A** = True   **B** = False   **C** = True   **D** = False   **E** = True

The commonest cell changes seen in non- or sublethal cell injury include increase in cell volume and accumulation of intracellular fat. The increase in volume is partly due to interference in the Na^+K^+ ATPase pump. Causes of fat accumulation include excess formation or entry or reduced dispersal. Excess formation may be seen in hypoxia, where free fatty acids are not oxidized to carbon dioxide, or starvation and diabetes, where there are increased free fatty acid levels in blood. It may even be due to cell poisons. Reduced fat dispersal may be due to lack of phospholipids leading to accumulation of globular fat, or lack of protein stabilized fat (fatty livers seen in kwashiorkor) or even excessive levels of cholesterol that antagonize the normal emulsifying functions of phospholipids.

Pyknosis is an old term that describes cell death and degeneration in which the nucleus shrinks, condenses and stains more deeply basophilic. The shrunken nucleus may progress on to breakage and fragmentation, which is known as karyorrhexis.

Heterolysis describes lysis of cells by enzymes derived from other cell types. Autolysis describes self-lysis of a cell by enzymes released by its lysosome.

Apoptosis describes programmed cell death, during which in two stages the cell is seen to separate from neighbouring cells and then fragment into membrane-bound components that either dissipate or are phagocytosed. The cell is seen to shrink, followed by condensation and aggregation of chromatin. Cytoplasmic blebs and 'apoptotic bodies' of membrane-bound fragments are then seen. These are usually phagocytosed.

Necrosis describes death of an area of an organ or tissue in which nearby tissue is preserved. The dead tissue may be classified either due to the cause of death or its appearance.

Aseptic necrosis describes death of part of a bone as a result of ischaemia; for example, aseptic necrosis of the head of femur as a result of femoral neck fracture. Coagulative, caseous and colliquative necrosis describe the appearances of the dead tissue.

In contrast to necrosis, apoptosis does not cause surrounding inflammation and occurs in tissue before any histological evidence is present.

3 **A** = True **B** = True **C** = True **D** = False **E** = True

Cell injury can be described anatomically in terms of pathology in the nucleus, cell membrane, enzymes or lysosomes. Acquired causes include harmful agents acting directly or being produced by metabolism, or indirect action such as enzyme interference (binding, denaturing or competitive inhibition). Direct action includes nitrogen mustards that combine with DNA and RNA and nitrosamines that alkylate by methylating DNA and RNA.

Examples of toxicity after metabolism includes methanol that is converted to formaldehyde by ethanol-metabolizing enzymes in the liver. Indirect action by interference with enzymes describes how cyanide binds with iron in cytochrome oxidase, thus inhibiting metabolism.

Injury to the nucleus includes injury to DNA either by mutation, breaks or transformations or by defective repair such as xeroderma pigmentosa where epithelial cells of skin lack UV specific endonucleases. These help to break abnormal dimer formation by UV-light, and so assist other enzymes to excise and repair damage to DNA.

As X-ray damage results in chain breakage of DNA, cells in xeroderma pigmentosa are able to repair damage due to X-ray exposure but are not able to repair UV damage.

Free radicals are molecules with a single unpaired electron in the outer orbit. They can be produced due to radiation energy, hypoxia and toxic agents such as carbon tetrachloride. They cause damage to cell membranes.

4 **A** = True **B** = True **C** = True **D** = True **E** = True

Leukotriene B_4, complement C5a, Il-1, TNF and IL-8, as well as the leukotrienes HPETE and HETE and platelet-activating factor are chemotactic agents for granulocytes.

Complement C3a is an anaphylotoxin that mainly causes increased vascular permeability but also has weak chemotactic properties. C5a is a chemotactic factor for neutrophils.

5 **A** = True **B** = True **C** = True **D** = True **E** = True **F** = False

Chemical mediators that cause increased vascular permeability include platelet-activating factor, kinins, lysosomal cationic proteins, histamine, complement C3a and C5a and leukotrienes C_4, D_4 and E_4.

6 **A** = True **B** = True **C** = False **D** = False **E** = True **F** = True

Chemical mediators directly causing vasodilation include nitric oxide (also known endothelial-derived relaxation factor) producing vasodilation locally by activating guanylyl cyclase after release from vascular endothelium and macrophages, prostaglandins I_2, E and E_2, kinins and histamine.

Interleukin-1 and bacterial endotoxin release may result in vasodilation by activation of neutrophils and mast cells causing release of vasoactive substances such as histamine.

7 **A** = True   **B** = True   **C** = True   **D** = False   **E** = True   **F** = True   **G** = True

Interleukin 1 is a cytokine. In common with other cytokines it is a low molecular weight protein involved in immunity and inflammation, whereby it plays a key role in influencing amplitude and duration of response. It is produced briefly around the site of inflammation and acts at very low concentrations by interacting with specific cell surface receptors. IL-1 is mainly produced by macrophages and acts in a positive-feedback manner on macrophages to increase IL-1 production.

IL-1 affects the immune system by stimulating B and T lymphocyte activation as well as natural killer cell activation and lymphokine production. Effects on granulocytes and mast cells include chemotaxis, degranulation, thromboxane production and histamine release. Effects on endothelium include increased leukocyte adhesion, platelet-activation factor production, prostaglandin I_2 (PGI_2) and PGE_2 and coagulation cascade activity. Effects on bone include increased reabsorption by osteoclast activity. Collagenase activity in the synovium as well as proteinase secretion in cartilage is also increased.

Metabolic effects of IL-1 include increased acute-phase protein production and decreased albumin synthesis by hepatocytes. A fall in cytochrome p450 activity is also seen.

Effects on the central nervous system include alteration in prostaglandin synthesis affecting the hypothalamus, resulting in fever. For this reason IL-1 is known as an endogenous pyrogen. It also causes a rise in ACTH levels.

In general, the effects of IL-1 include a fall in systemic vascular resistance, mean blood pressure and central venous pressure. Heart rate and cardiac output are seen to increase.

8 **A** = True   **B** = True   **C** = False   **D** = False   **E** = True   **F** = False

Phagocytosis is essentially a function of neutrophils and macrophages. Eosinophils are granulocytes with acid-staining (eosinophilic) granules that also play a phagocytic role. They attack parasites that are too large to be successfully destroyed by phagocytosis and release chemical mediators including leukotriene C_4 and platelet-activating factor that increase vascular permeability and are chemotactic. Circulating eosinophil levels are often raised in allergic conditions.

Basophils have basophilic granules and are similar in many ways to mast cells. They contain and release histamine and heparin as well as other chemical mediators when activated. Basophils and mast cells play an important role in type I hypersensitivity.

9 **A** = True **B** = True **C** = True **D** = True **E** = False

Mast cell degranulation leads to release of primary mediators (preformed) and second-ary mediators (synthesied and then released). Primary mediators include histamine, adenosine, eosinophil and neutrophil chemotactic factors, hydrolytic enzymes that facilitate kinin and complement production and heparin. Secondary mediators include products of arachidonic acid via the lypoxygenase pathway (leukotrienes, especially B_4, C_4, D_4, E_4) and via the cyclooxygenase pathway (prostaglandins, especially D_2), platelet-activating factor and cytokines including TNF-α, IL-1, IL-3, IL-4, IL-5 and IL-6.

10 **A** = False **B** = True **C** = False **D** = False **E** = True

Acute inflammation is defined as the immediate response to tissue insult resulting in the 'cardinal' signs of 'rubor' (redness), 'calor' (heat), 'tumour' (swelling), 'dolor' (pain) and 'functio laesa' (loss of function). It is characterized by vascular and cellular events. One of the early vascular events is relaxation of arterioles due to local release of chemical mediators, and it has been shown that denervation still allows this response to take place in the presence of local injury and inflammation. Opsonins such IgG and C3b coat bacteria or foreign particles in order that they are recognized as foreign. This process is known as opsonization and prepares neutrophils and macrophages better for phagocytosis.

Interleukin 1 is produced by activated macrophages. Interleukin 2 is produced by activated T lymphocytes and acts to stimulate T cell activation as well as differentiation in proliferation. Increased vascular permeability in the first 30 min of inflammation occurs due to endothelial cell contraction leaving gaps. This only affects 20–60 μm venules and not capillaries or arterioles. It is usually due to the effect of histamine release.

In vitro, it has been shown that between 4 and 6 h there is endothelial retraction, resulting in gaps. This is due to cytoskeletal reorganization separating endothelial cells. It is cytokine mediated and is due to release of IL-1, TNF and IFN α.

Direct endothelial injury resulting in cell death and separation causes an immediate sustained response involving venules, capillaries and arterioles. Leakage is seen to begin immediately and lasts for hours. The delayed response is characterized by a 2–12 h delay which lasts 5 h to days and this involves capillaries as well. It is seen to be caused by thermal injury, X-ray or UV radiation (sunburn). The mechanism is unclear. The immediate transient response is due to mild injury.

11 **A** = True **B** = False **C** = False **D** = True **E** = True **F** = True

Chronic inflammation describes an outcome of acute inflammation progressing for weeks or months. Three main processes of active inflammation, marked tissue destruc-tion and healing are seen. Due to the chronicity, chronic inflammation has histological differences to acute inflammation. Neutrophils do not play a large role. In contrast, mononuclear cells such as macrophages, plasma cells and lymphocytes are seen. Products of these cells result in collagen and tissue destruction.

Repair is seen by the presence of fibroblasts producing collagen (and possibly fibrosis) and new proliferating blood vessels sprouting from existing vessels into the immature collagen. The appearance of buds of new vessels amidst the fibroblasts and collagen gives the appearance of pink, soft granular tissue. This is thus referred to as 'granulation tissue'.

The presence of the plasma cell is a reliable sign of chronicity. It produces antibodies that act locally against the foreign antigen.

The half-life of a monocyte is approximately 22–24 h. Tissue macrophages, however, last for months.

Granulomatous inflammation is a specialized form of chronic inflammation indicated by the presence of a granuloma, which is defined by the presence of three or more macrophage-derived cells. Macrophages are derived from blood monocytes and although relatively inactive, they retain the ability for division. Macrophages activate and transform to epithelioid cells (with an epithelial-like appearance) or may fuse in the centre of granulomas forming multinucleated giant cells (Langhans' giant cells). The T cell-mediated immune reaction is also a feature of granulomatous inflammation as this is required in the activation of macrophages.

12 **A** = False   **B** = False   **C** = True   **D** = False   **E** = True   **F** = True   **G** = True

Interferons are cytokines that may be classified into three groups: α, β and γ. Interferon-α is produced mainly by infected leukocytes; interferon-β is produced by fibroblasts, and interferon-γ is produced by activated T lymphocytes.

Although production may be stimulated by bacterial cell wall lypopolysaccharide, the strongest stimulus for synthesis is double-stranded RNA virus (often produced as an intermediate step in viral replication). Functions of interferon include inhibition of viral replication. Although there is no single method, the main mechanism is by 'inducing' certain protein kinases whose synthesis would then be switched on by contact with double-stranded viral RNA. Protein kinases phosphorylate translator proteins and so translation of mRNA is seen to be inhibited. Protein synthesis is also inhibited by activation of other proteins.

Interferon is specific for a particular species, and is not virus specific.

Other functions of interferon include induction of fever and interferon-γ is particularly effective in activating macrophages and increasing expression of cell surface antigens associated with either class I or class II MHC molecules.

13 **A** = False   **B** = True   **C** = True   **D** = True   **E** = False

The complement system describes an innate non-specific form of immunity created by an enzyme cascade used to destroy microbes or to attract and activate phagocytes against antigens. It consists of a classical and alternative pathway. The antibody-dependent classical pathway requires two or more IgG or IgM antibodies bound to a microbe to trigger the cascade via formation of a C1qrs complex. The alternative pathway describes how the most abundant circulatory complement protein, C3, is split after contact with microbial polysaccharides, directly leading to production of its cleavage products.

C3b binds to the microbe acting as an opsonin and C3a is released. These events lead to the common pathway of the production of the C5b-9 membrane attack complex as well as chemotactic agents, mediators increasing vascular permeability and opsonins.

14 **A** = True   **B** = True   **C** = True   **D** = True   **E** = True

Acute-phase proteins are proteins that increase in concentration during the acute-phase response (infection, inflammation or tissue damage). Their role is important locally and systemically. Activation of the coagulation and fibrinolytic pathways sees a rise in fibrinogen, prothrombin, factor VIII and plasminogen levels.

Heat-labile complement proteins produced by the liver and whose serum levels rise during the acute-phase response include C1s, C2, C3, C4, C5 and C9. Raised levels of α_1-antitrypsin and other proteinase inhibitors are seen, as are raised levels of transport proteins, including caeruloplasmin and ferritin. Among a group of proteins with a non-specific or local role, C-reactive protein, serum amyloid A protein and fibronectin levels are seen to rise.

15 **A** = True   **B** = False   **C** = True   **D** = False   **E** = False

Hypersensitivity is described as an exaggerated immune response causing tissue damage. Type I hypersensitivity is an immediate hypersensitivity, also known as allergy. It has an early and late phase in response to an allergen.

The early phase known as a 'flare and weal' reaction, occurs within 20 min, primarily due to mast cell mediators. This phase may be inhibited by drugs such as sodium chromoglycate, which can bind to different mast cell receptors, stabilizing them and making the mast cell resistant to activation.

A late phase seen after 5 h and lasting for up to 24 h is often seen following a large immediate response. This is characterized by dense cellular infiltrates and more oedema than before. It is thought to be due to neutrophil chemotactic factor released by the mast cells. Corticosteroids are found to be useful in blocking this late phase.

The underlying cellular mechanism of type I hypersensitivity begins by contact of antigen with antigen-presenting cells (APCs) such as tissue macrophages. Antigen-presenting cells induce T helper cell stimulation which results in production of inter-leukins such as IL-5 (eosinophil activation) and IL-4, which induces specific B cell 'class switching' to produce IgE antibodies locally.

IgE binding to mast cells and cross-linking of mast cell IgE receptors results in mast cell degranulation and release of chemical mediators, both stored and synthesized *de novo.* IgE is a large molecule and almost all is tissue bound. Very little is found in the circulation. Raised serum IgE levels at rest are associated with atopy. Systemic anaphylaxis is a result of massive IgE release into the circulation binding on to tissue mast cells located around small blood vessels throughout the body and circulating basophils. Histamine released into the circulation causes peripheral vasodilation and increased capillary permeability.

16 **A** = True   **B** = False   **C** = True   **D** = True   **E** = True

Type II hypersensitivity is also known as 'antigen–antibody-dependent cytotoxicity'. It describes antigen binding of IgM or IgG to activate complement via the classical pathway or facilitate phagocytosis via the Fc receptor on neutrophils, macrophages and eosinophils. This mechanism is referred to as hypersensitivity when the immune response is inappropriate or exaggerated and results in tissue damage.

It may be classified as either isoimmune or autoimmune depending on whether the antigen belongs to a member of the same species or belongs to the subject themselves. Examples of isoimmune hypersensitivity include incompatible blood transfusion reactions (antibodies to ABO or rhesus antigens on transfused red cells), rhesus incompatibility and haemolytic disease of the newborn as well as hyperacute organ transplant rejection (preformed circulating antibodies to the donor organ). Note that acute transplant rejection is a cell-mediated type IV hypersensitivity reaction that occurs between 7 and 90 days after transplant.

Examples of autoimmune type II hypersensitivity include autoimmune haemolytic anaemia, autoimmune thrombocytopenia, myasthenia gravis (antibodies against the muscle motor end-plate acetylcholine receptor) and Goodpasture's syndrome (IgG antibodies against basement membrane, especially those of kidney and lungs).

The Coomb's test is a means of detecting red cells coated with antibodies by making them agglutinate through the addition of albumin or serum containing immunoglobulins against the coating antibodies. It is positive in detecting rhesus antibodies as well as red cell antibodies found in autoimmune haemolytic anaemia.

17 **A** = True   **B** = False   **C** = True   **D** = True   **E** = True

Type III hypersensitivity involves persistent immune antigen/antibody complex formation with deposition of insoluble complexes at particular sites, resulting in an acute inflammatory reaction. Three basic events are complement activation, influx of polymorphs and platelet aggregation. Complement activation results along with complement-mediated tissue damage, anaphylotoxin release, and release of mast cell mediators. This results in an influx of polymorphs that attempt to phagocytose the immune complexes and during this process release their contents causing further tissue damage. Platelet aggregation is also seen and this provides further vasoactive amine release as well as causing local ischaemia as a result of the formation of microthrombi. Examples include immune complex glomerulonephritis (build-up of large granules containing antigen, immunoglobulin and complement C3), serum sickness (injection of large doses of foreign serum resulting in a reaction up to 8 days later) and Arthus reaction (injection of antigen intradermally in an immunized subject; can be blocked by depleting complement or polymorphs).

18 **A** = False   **B** = True   **C** = False   **D** = True   **E** = True

Type IV hypersensitivity describes delayed-type hypersensitivity via a T cell-dependent cell-mediated immune response. T cells express the T cell receptor complex made up of a heterodimeric T cell receptor (TCR) and the CD3 complex (exclusive to T cells). As a further differentiation, these cells either express CD4 or CD8 receptors, classifying them as CD4 (T4) or CD8 (T8) cells. The CD (cluster of differentiation) molecule describes a family of cell surface markers identified by monoclonal antibodies.

The CD4 (T4) cell is associated with the term 'T helper cell' and by the production of cytokines. It influences T and B cell response and in particular can induce the cytotoxic function of the CD8 (T8) cell. It recognizes antigens restricted to class II of the major histocompatibility complex.

The CD8 (T8) cell is associated with the term 'T cytotoxic cell' and is destructive by direct cytotoxicity. It recognizes antigens restricted to class I of the major histocompatibility complex.

The major histocompatibility complex is a gene locus located on the short arm of chromosome 6. There are two classes located here: class I which expresses human leukocyte antigens (A-, B- and C-) on all nucleated cells and class II (HLA-DP, -DQ and -DR) which expresses antigens on antigen-presenting cells (APCs) and is thus found on macrophages, dendritic cells (and Langerhans' cells) and B cells. Class I antigens are essential to activate T cytotoxic cells and class II antigens must be present to activate T helper cells.

The sequence of events begins with a foreign antigen entering either an APC or (in the case of a virus) any nucleated cell. Part of the foreign antigen is expressed as a hapten on either the class I or class II human leukocyte surface antigen. This activates either T cytotoxic cells or T helper cells. T helper cells differentiate and, in the process, release cytokines (interleukins and interferons) that influence B cell proliferation and differentiation and specific antibody production, as well as activating natural killer cells, macrophages and granulocytes.

Activation of T cytotoxic cells results in direct cytotoxicity by cell binding and enzyme release, including 'perforin' to destroy cell membranes. Its most important role is in the elimination of virally infected nucleated cells (class I antigenic). T cytotoxic cells may also activate macrophages.

Type IV hypersensitivity is an exaggerated cell-mediated immune response causing tissue damage. It takes longer than 12 h (usually 48–72 h) to develop and involves previously sensitized T helper cell activation. It is characterized by erythema and induration and a heavy mononuclear and lymphocytic infiltration. This may progress to granuloma formation where epithelioid cells and other macrophage-derived cells are seen.

Cytokines released include IL-2, IFN γ and macrophage and lymphocytic chemotactic and activation factors by T cells. Macrophages release cytokines including IL-1, IL-6 and IL-8 as well as TNF. As T cells only recognize haptens expressed by their own class I and II human leukocyte antigens, type IV hypersensitivity cannot be transferred by serum to non-sensitized subjects.

Examples of type IV hypersensitivity include the Mantoux and Heaf (tuberculin) skin test for tuberculosis, the lepromin test for leprosy and contact dermatitis.

19 **A** = False   **B** = True   **C** = False   **D** = False   **E** = True

The cornea is in a privileged site for transplantation due to its lack of vascularization. For this reason, preoperative HLA matching is not essential. Corneal grafting usually involves transplantation of an allograft (from a different member of the same species). An isograft refers to donor tissue from a genetically identical individual (twins, HLA-identical siblings). Transplant of a xenograft describes living donor tissue between species.

Types of immune rejection may be classified as hyperacute, humoral, acute and chronic.

Hyperacute rejection may occur within minutes or hours of transplant and is a humoral-mediated rejection due to preformed antibodies involving complement and occurs usually in association with xenograft transplants. It is not usually a problem with allograft transplantation and requires serological cross-matching in order to minimize its risk.

Acute rejection is usually seen after a week and may not occur until 3–4 months after transplant. It is a cell-mediated immune response in a host not previously sensitized. It is mainly associated with allograft transplantation and involves CD4 (T helper) and CD8 (T cytotoxic) cells mediating a mononuclear–macrophage response. (A small humoral component may also been seen in the form of vasculitis.)

Chronic rejection is a vascular rejection with a poorly understood mechanism occurring usually after three months (even as late as 10 years) in association with allografts. Inflammatory atheroma-like occlusion of the vascular intima is seen with dense intimal fibrosis resulting in secondary ischaemia of the graft.

Major attention has been directed towards acute rejection. In the past, the phenomenon of tolerance was explained by the fact that T cells were only activated if they recognized foreign antigens in combination with one's own MHC molecules. It has been shown, however, that donor allograft dendritic cells ('passenger leucocytes') react to cells expressed by foreign MHC molecules and facilitate a host-cell-mediated immune response. Passenger leucocytes recognize class II MHC molecules of the graft and present to host T cells. These class II molecules are found on donor cells and more importantly, vascular endothelium, and are usually expressed following the trauma of surgery. Following recognition, the passenger leucocytes act as antigen-presenting cells themselves and trigger CD4 (T helper) cells to activate a cell-mediated immune response. Cytokines released (e.g. IL-2) stimulate CD8 (T cytotoxic) cell proliferation and maturation, and macrophage-activating factors facilitate activation of macrophages. The result is an interstitial mononuclear/macrophage cellular infiltrate and lysis of allogenic cells. Lymphokines such as IFN-β and TNF-β activate macrophages. IL-4, IL-5 and IL-6 are required for B cell activation to produce antigraft antibodies.

Cyclosporin A is a T cell-specific fungal peptide that revolutionized transplant surgery in the 1980s by its ability to cause specific immunosuppression. It selectively penetrates CD4 (T helper) cells and interferes with division, maturation and production of these cells. It also reduces production of IL-2 as well as sensitivity to IL-2 (by reduction of IL-2 receptor expression). Its main side-effects are nephrotoxicity and hepatotoxicity as well as the increased risk of lymphomas associated with Epstein–Barr virus.

20 **A** = False **B** = True **C** = True **D** = True **E** = False

Atherosclerosis is a disease of large and medium-sized muscular arteries (coronary, cerebral and popliteal) and elastic vessels (aorta, carotid, iliac). The lesion consists of a raised intimal plaque with a lipid core and a fibrous cap. It may be associated with smooth muscle cells and macrophages (often fat filled) as well as a cell-mediated immune reaction surrounding it.

The current theory is of a response to endothelial injury resulting in intimal thickening. Exposure of subendothelial collagen attracts platelet deposition and initiates a repair process evidenced by the release of platelet growth factors, the most important being platelet-derived growth factor (PDGF) (trophic to smooth muscle cells in the intima and chemotactic for fibroblasts, smooth muscle cells, macrophages and neutrophils), along with endothelial growth factors such as TNF, transforming growth factor β (TGF-β) and interferons γ.

Intimal smooth muscle cell proliferation is seen and fatty streaks develop. The resultant intimal thickening due to proliferation is associated with lipid deposition, extracellular matrix (proteoglycan), elastic tissue and fibrous tissue (collagen).

Plaques may be classified as type I (smooth or stable) and type II (cracked or unstable). The type II plaque is seen to be the preceding event to sudden thrombosis and plaque occlusion. It has a partly unknown pathogenesis but is characterized by inflammation, foamy (fat-filled) macrophages and smooth muscle cells. The 'cracking' and exposure of exquisitely thrombogenic connective tissue results in platelet aggregation and is followed by triggering of the clotting cascade, resulting in thrombosis and occlusion.

Complication of plaque formation thus includes ulceration, thrombosis, intraplaque haemorrhage, calcification and aneurysm formation.

Aneurysm formation is due to the thickened intimal layer resulting in thinning and loss of smooth muscle cells in the underlying media layer. This layer dilates locally as a result of the overlying plaque atheroma.

The main factors associated with atherosclerosis are hyperlipidaemia, in particular, hypercholesterolaemia (raised LDL, reduced HDL), hypertension, smoking and diabetes.

21 **A** = False   **B** = True   **C** = True   **D** = True   **E** = True   **F** = True   **G** = True   **H** = True

A thrombus is a solid mass formed in the heart, arteries, veins or capillaries from circulating components of blood. According to Virchow's triad, the risk factors for thrombus may be classified as changes in the intimal surface of vessels, changes in blood flow and changes in the constituents of blood.

Changes in the intimal surface of vessels include atherosclerosis, injury, inflammation (temporal arteritis, polyarteritis nodosa) and tumour invasion.

Changes in blood flow include the speed (stasis and venous thrombosis) and type of flow (turbulent flow causing cardiac and arterial thrombi).

Changes in the constituents of blood leading to a hypercoagulant state may be classified as congenital or acquired. Congenital causes include antithrombin III deficiency, protein C deficiency, protein S deficiency and mutation in coagulation factor V (factor V Leiden) or activated protein C resistance.

Acquired causes may be divided into high and low risk. High-risk factors include prolonged bedrest and immobilization, myocardial infarction, tissue trauma (including surgery, burns, fractures), cardiac failure (stasis), acute leukaemia, cancer (release of factor X or extrinsic pathway-activating products), myeloproliferative disorders, DIC (disseminated intravascular coagulation) and homocystinuria (toxic to endothelium). Low-risk factors include the oral contraceptive pill and increased levels of plasma fibrinogen, prothrombin and factors VII, VIII and X, atrial fibrillation, hyperlipidaemia, sickle cell anaemia (occlusion causing secondary stasis), smoking and thrombocytosis.

22 **A** = True   **B** = False   **C** = True   **D** = True   **E** = True

Infarction is a large localized area of ischaemic necrosis within a tissue or organ either due to arterial insufficiency or venous occlusion. The majority are due to thromboembolic arterial occlusion.

It may be pale in the case of arterial occlusion, especially in solid tissue, or haemorrhagic in venous occlusion or tissue previously congested. 'Infarct' implies 'stuffed' with blood from surrounding tissue. Histologically, most infarcts tend to be wedge-shaped with the apex pointing to the origin of vascular occlusion.

Initial events include no cellular change until the first few hours, after which the area becomes poorly defined and darker in colour. Over 24 h, definition improves and the colour becomes darker. Between 24 and 36 h, the blood extrudes, leaving the tissue area paler. A narrow red margin reveals an inflammatory response with neutrophils followed by macrophages, cellular infiltrate and a fibroblastic repair process preserving the outer margins.

In the brain, dead tissue undergoes liquefactive necrosis, cavity formation and is replaced by glial tissue synthesized by astrocytes. Elsewhere in the body the dead tissue undergoes coagulative necrosis. In the presence of a bacterial infection around the area of necrosis, abscess formation is seen. Factors determining the risk of infarction include the nature of the arterial supply and venous drainage (end-artery or dual circulation, anastomosis, single or dual venous drainage), rate of onset of occlusion and the type of tissue and its vulnerability to ischaemia.

23 **A** = False   **B** = True   **C** = True   **D** = True   **E** = True

Oedema refers to excess fluid in the extracellular space. It may be in exudate (including purulent exudate) or transudate. *Exudate* is cellular containing high levels of protein, especially plasma proteins (including fibrinogen) and has a raised specific gravity (1.020). *Transudate* may contain a few cells and low levels of protein (1 g/100 ml) mainly albumin. Specific gravity is less than 1.012.

Pulmonary oedema may be haemodynamic in origin (with increased hydrostatic pressure, reduced oncotic pressure or lymphatic obstruction) or microvascular in origin. This may be due to infectious agents, inhalation of gases, aspiration, drugs, shock, trauma or sepsis, radiation or in severe acute pancreatitis. It is also seen in association with acutely raised intracranial pressure (neurogenic origin) and is occasionally seen at high altitudes.

Filariasis is a disease caused by a nematode worm (*Wuchereria bancrofti*) found in groin lymphatics. On dying, the nematode can elicit a local inflammatory reaction resulting in lymphatic obstruction and oedema of the external genitalia and lower limbs.

Hypoalbuminaemia results in fluid shift from the intravascular to interstitial space. Due to a resulting fall in plasma volume, there is a fall in renal perfusion that stimulates renin–angiotensin release and so results in a secondary hyperaldosteronism. Due to a basic protein deficiency, however, any salt and water retained will inevitably leave the intravascular space to enter the interstitial space as oedema.

24 **A** = True   **B** = False   **C** = False   **D** = True   **E** = False

Pigmentation may be exogenous (carbon, tattoos) or endogenous (lipofuscin, bilirubin, melanin, haemosiderin). Lipofuscin is an insoluble 'wear and tear' pigment made of lipid polymers and proteins. They are formed as a result of lipid peroxidation of membranes and indicate free radical activity. In themselves they are not toxic. They are yellowy brown in colour, they are found in the heart and liver and are also seen beneath the retinal pigment epithelium as a result of pigment epithelium breakdown and photoreceptor renewal.

Haemosiderin is formed by iron accumulation either from ferritin or haemoglobin and may be local or systemic. The best example of local haemosiderosis is a bruise. By the action of macrophage and lysosomal enzymes the dark red/blue colour of haemoglobin transforms to dark green/blue (biliverdin) and then bilirubin. The later golden yellow colour of haemosiderin is due to iron deposition remaining. Raised levels of bilirubin in the conjunctival vessels during jaundice give rise to the yellow appearance of the sclera. This is not due to scleral protein binding.

One of the key steps in melanin metabolism involves conversion of tyrosine to DOPA. Tyrosine is also broken down along with phenylalanine by the enzyme homogentisic acid oxidase. Deficiency of this enzyme and build-up of homogentisic acid causes dark brown pigmentation of the skin and eyes (ochronosis) and is known as alcaptonuria.

25 **A** = True   **B** = False   **C** = False   **D** = True   **E** = False   **F** = True

Heterotrophic calcification describes deposition of calcium outside bone and enamel. It may be dystrophic or metastatic.

Dystrophic calcification is found in the presence of normal serum calcium levels in areas of necrosis, atherosclerosis, tuberculosis or haematoma (not old cerebral hae-matoma which undergoes reabsorption). It may be seen on aortic stenotic valves. Calcium deposition may be intracellular in the mitochondria of dead cells, or extracellular. Psammoma bodies are lamellae of dystrophic calcification around necrotic cells. These are often seen in intracranial tumours.

Metastatic calcification occurs in normal tissue in the presence of hypercalcaemia. Hypercalcaemia may be due to bone reabsorption, increased gut absorption or as a result of raised serum phosphate levels due to renal osteodystrophy. Causes therefore include hyperparathyroidism, increased levels of vitamin D, sarcoidosis, hyperthyroidism and bone malignancy (metastatic disease, myeloma). Calcium deposition is seen in kidney tubules, lungs (alveolar walls), gastric mucosa, coronary arteries and the cornea.

26 **A** = False   **B** = True   **C** = True   **D** = True   **E** = True   **F** = True

To quote Sir Rupert Willis: 'A neoplasm is an abnormal mass of tissue, the growth of which exceeds and is unco-ordinated with that of the normal tissues and persist in the same excessive manner after cessation of the stimuli which evoked the change.' This implies an abnormal autonomous proliferation, differentiation and relationship with surrounding tissue. A 'tumour' is a swelling that may or may not be neoplastic, although today, the term tumour is usually taken to be synonymous with neoplasm.

Benign neoplasms are well differentiated and grow slowly in an expansile non-invasive manner with very few cells undergoing mitosis. They do not metastasize.

Malignant neoplasms are less differentiated with a high rate of cell turnover. They display both cellular and nuclear pleomorphism with variations in both cellular and nuclear size and shape. The nuclei are also hyperchromatic with a large amount of DNA and dark staining. Rather than the normal 1:4 to 1:6 nuclear: cytoplasmic ratio, there is an increased nuclear: cytoplasmic ratio of up to 1:1. There is also loss of normal ploidy.

Malignant neoplasms may spread locally in an invasive manner or by lymphatics, blood or across a cavity such as the peritoneum. Although mortality is associated with malignancy, benign neoplasms can result in fatal local mechanical effects as in the case of benign neoplasms of the brain, resulting in hydrocephalus and raised intracranial pressure.

27 **A** = False   **B** = False   **C** = True   **D** = False   **E** = False

Dysplasia refers to the loss or reduction in the degree of differentiation of cell types, especially epithelial cells, without invasion of surrounding tissues. Dysplastic cells show pleomorphism, hyperchromatic nuclei and evidence of mitosis appearing not only in the basal layers. Although it is commonly seen before malignant neoplasia, dysplasia does not always progress and is reversible in the presence of moderate change not involving the full epithelial thickness. Dysplasia of all epithelial layers but not invading the basement membrane is referred to as carcinoma *in situ*.

A hamartoma is a non-neoplastic congenital malformation that forms a neoplastic-like mass, but grows at a normal rate (unlike neoplasms) to its surrounding tissue without a capsule and often regresses with age. Examples include port–wine stains and Peutz-Jeghers polyps.

Metaplasia describes the change from one fully differentiated form of tissue to another fully differentiated form. Examples include Barrett's oesophagus, where the normal squamous epithelium lining the oesophagus is replaced by columnar epithelium due to persistent damage as a result of reflux oesophagitis, and tobacco-induced metaplasia of the bronchus where normal pseudostratified ciliated columnar epithelium of the bronchus is replaced by squamous epithelium.

A polyp is a pedunculated mass arising from an epithelial surface as a result of neoplasia, hamartoma (non-neoplastic), inflammation or metaplasia.

28 **A** = False   **B** = True   **C** = True   **D** = True   **E** = False   **F** = False

The normal cell cycle is made up of a G_1, S, G_2 and M phase. The G_1 phase has a variable length of days to years, the other phases are reasonably constant.

When in the G_1 phase (also known as the 'gap' phase) the cell may enter a resting G_0 phase, or opt out and terminally differentiate to eventually die. It leaves the G_1 phase after passing the restriction point late in G_1, where it is thought that synthesis of DNA polymerase begins. The cell then enters the S phase (up to 12 h) of DNA synthesis and following a short G_2 phase (up to 6 h) enters the M (mitosis) phase (up to 2 h).

Hyperplasia refers to a stimulus-led increase in the number of cells of an organ. It may be physiological or pathological. Hyperplasia is seen in hormonal stimulation of endocrine glands such as the adrenal and thyroid glands. Negative feedback regulation of the hormonal signal controls the degree of hyperplasia.

Pathological hyperplasia with the example of endometrial proliferation is associated with an increased risk of developing endometrial carcinoma, particularly if there is associated dysplasia.

Hypertrophy is a demand-led increase in cell size of an organ with no increase in the number. The increase in size is due to an increase in synthesis of structural components. Increase in cell size due to cellular swelling or oedema is not described as hypertrophy.

29 **A** = False   **B** = True   **C** = True   **D** = True   **E** = False

Tumour spread may be direct, lymphatic, bloodborne or metastatic. Direct spread involves detachment. This requires loss of cell-to-cell adhesiveness. A reduction in cell surface fibronectin is seen to reduce cell-to-cell binding. A loss of anchorage dependence is seen. Progressive infiltration, invasion and destruction of surrounding tissue is seen. Invasion of basement membrane and extracellular matrix requires attachment to and degradation of the matrix. Increased cell surface expression of the laminin receptor is needed in order to bind basement membrane laminin. Tumour cells either secrete or induce secretion of proteolytic enzymes. The three classes involved are serine proteinases, cysteine proteinases and metalloproteinases.

Type IV collagenase is a metalloproteinase that is very important during invasion in cleaving basement membrane.

Tumour angiogenesis is crucial for tumour growth and spread. The most powerful and important tumour-derived angiogenic factors include the fibroblast growth factors (FGFs), which are chemotactic and mitogenic for endothelial cells and stimulate proteolytic enzymes to facilitate stromal infiltration of new vessels, TGFα and β, EGF and PDGF.

30 **A** = True   **B** = False   **C** = True   **D** = True   **E** = False   **F** = True

A carcinogen is an environmental agent, either physical, chemical or viral, responsible for either the initiation or promotion of malignant transformation. Initiation is a result of exposure to a carcinogen whose active form binds on to DNA and irreversibly initiates a change. Promotion occurs following possibly repeated exposures to non-mutagenic irritants that result in progression of carcinogenesis. Chemical carcinogens include direct-acting alkylating agents, polycyclic aromatic hydrocarbons (skin cancer), aromatic amines and azo dyes (bladder cancer, by liver detoxification and further breakdown by the enzyme glucuronidase in the bladder), saccharine (bladder cancer in rats) and asbestos (carcinoma of the bronchus, mesothelioma and cancer of the gastrointestinal tract).

Physical carcinogens include ionizing radiation which predisposes to leukaemia (except chronic lymphocytic leukaemia) and thyroid carcinoma (in the young) and ultraviolet radiation. UV-B is most implicated in skin cancer. UV-C is perhaps more carcinogenic but is absorbed by the ozone layer and UV-A has a photosensitizing effect, but has been shown to cause cancer in animals.

Included in the viral carcinogens is the human papillomavirus, especially types 16 and 18 (however, types 31, 33 and 35 may also be factors) which have been implicated in carcinoma of the cervix. HPV-6 and 11 are associated with genital warts and are considered a 'low risk' for malignancy.

31 A = True **B** = True **C** = True **D** = True **E** = True

Normal cell signalling is transient and in response to a stimulus. It usually consists of a growth factor binding to a membrane receptor which signals an intracellular secondary messenger transducer protein to interact with a nuclear receptor and this increases production or expression of DNA.

A proto-oncogene is a normal cell-signalling DNA sequence that codes for anything from the growth factor to enzymes produced by upregulation of DNA. An oncogene is a mutated-cell signalling gene that encodes a step in the cell-signalling pathway. Oncogenes are either overexpressed or remain active regardless of stimulus cessation.

The *erb*B oncogene codes for the EGF cell membrane receptor; the *ras* oncogene codes for the secondary messenger G protein; the *myc* and *fos* oncogenes code for nuclear regulating proteins. The *sis* oncogene codes for production of paracrine growth factors such as PDGF. Oncogenes may be carried by the virus genome. DNA oncogenic viruses include the papillomavirus, herpes viruses (EBV, Burkitt's lymphoma and nasopharyngeal carcinoma), and hepatitis B virus (hepatoma). Oncogenes may be activated by proto-oncogene overexpression such as gene amplification or excess promotion in the case of translocation of 8–*myc* proto-oncogene to chromosome 14 (the immunoglobulin chromosome), resulting in promotion of immunoglobulin production and Burkitt's lymphoma. Oncogenes may also be activated by alteration in their structure (point mutations etc.) or even by deletion or mutation of a suppressed gene.

32 A = True **B** = True **C** = False **D** = True **E** = False **F** = True

Tumour markers are substances present in the body in concentrations that may be related to the presence of a tumour. They may be either expressed or secreted and should be able to suggest tumour size and/or aggressiveness.

β-Human chromic gonadotrophin (βHCG) is raised in trophoblastic tumours as well as germ cell tumours. CEA (carcino-embryonic antigen) may be used to confirm the presence of colonic carcinomas. CA125 is raised in 90% of women with stage 3 or 4 ovarian cancer. PSA (prostate-specific antigen) is more sensitive than the previously used acid phosphatase in marking the presence and progress of prostatic carcinoma. Serum AFP (α-fetoprotein) is raised in over 50% of patients with hepatocellular carcinoma. CA15–3 is a mucin marker found in raised levels in the presence of breast carcinoma.

33 A = False **B** = True **C** = True **D** = True **E** = True **F** = True **G** = False

Amyloid is associated with a spectrum of diseases caused by the deposition of extracellular protein made up of β-pleated sheets. Amyloid is not a carbohydrate (as its name 'starch-like' would suggest) but is a protein which stains a rich brown colour with Lugol's iodine and shows yellow/green birefringence (dichroism) when bound with

Congo Red dye and viewed in polarized light. The main feature is of β-pleated fibril sheets.

Amyloidosis may be classified into either: (1) amyloidosis of immune origin (AL light chain type), or (2) reactive systemic amyloidosis.

The immune origin type is an acquired disorder characterized by monoclonal proliferation of B lymphocytes or plasma cells. This proliferation may be neoplastic as in the case of myeloma. The amyloid in this type is related to a light chain (especially γ type) or a terminal fragment produced that is then somehow converted from the normal α-helical structure to the characteristic β-pleated sheet structure. Antibodies raised against this protein have been found to also react with a similar light chain, the Bence-Jones protein. The immune origin amyloid is known to systemically deposit in organs and cause neuropathy, restrictive cardiomyopathy, skin nodules, polyarthropathy, carpal tunnel syndrome and macroglossia.

Reactive systemic amyloidosis is related to a liver-produced acute-phase protein known as the serum amyloid A (SAA) protein. This is a precursor to the amyloid which is derived by cleavage of 28 amino acid residues at the carboxy-terminal. Due to raised levels of SAA protein in inflammation, amyloid is seen to be deposited systemically in the presence of chronic inflammation, either due to infection or hypersensitivity. It is also seen in neoplasia. Deposition occurs in the spleen, liver and kidney (common cause of death due to chronic renal failure). In rare cases amyloid may be inherited in an autosomal dominant pattern with varying origins of the amyloid protein, one of which is the β protein. The β protein (also known as A4 protein) is deposited in the brain in Down's syndrome (and inherited Alzheimer's disease). The gene for this protein is found on the long arm of chromosome 21.

MICROBIOLOGY
Questions

1 The normal flora of the eyelids and conjunctiva includes

   A *Staphylococcus epidermidis*
   B Diphtheroids
   C *Staphylococcus aureus*
   D *Streptococcus pneumoniae*
   E *Candida albicans*

2 *Staphylococcus*

   A species are catalase positive
   B *saprophyticus* is coagulase negative
   C *epidermidis* is novobiocin sensitive
   D *aureus* is coagulase positive
   E *aureus* is an aerobic or facultative anaerobic organism

3 Which of the following statements about *Staphylococcus* are true?

   A Cross-infection is increased with penicillin resistance.
   B Cross-infection is due to colonies on curtains and linen.
   C *Staph. aureus* causes osteomyelitis.
   D *Staph. aureus* is a nasal and skin commensal.
   E Human carriers are more usually male than female.

4 *Staphylococcus aureus*

   A produces protein S
   B produces enterotoxins and haemolysins
   C is associated with endocarditis
   D grows on simple media
   E strains can be characterized by bacteriophage typing

5 Staphylococcal infections related to the eye include

  A blepharitis
  B conjunctivitis
  C ulcerative keratitis (corneal ulcer)
  D endophthalmitis
  E hordeolum and chalazion

6 Which of the following statements about streptococci are true?

  A Streptococci are catalase positive.
  B Streptococci are mostly facultative anaerobes.
  C Streptococci are classified using the Lancefield classification based on the presence of surface antigen M proteins.
  D Streptococci are never commensal.
  E Ninety per cent of streptococcal infections in humans are due to a β-haemolytic Lancefield group A organism.

7 *Streptococcus pyogenes*

  A is a commensal of the nose in up to 25% of the population
  B is a commensal of the throat in up to 4% of the population
  C is sensitive to bacitracin
  D can be subtyped by Griffiths typing
  E produces oxygen-stable streptolysin O

8 *Streptococcus pneumoniae* (pneumococcus)

  A is a β-haemolytic gram-positive ovoid diplococcus
  B is resistant to optochin
  C is an upper respiratory tract commensal
  D is lysed by bile
  E possesses 84 different types of antigenic capsules

9 *Streptococcus viridans* is responsible for

  A green colonies on blood agar
  B acute glomerulonephritis
  C subacute bacterial endocarditis
  D lobar pneumonia
  E rheumatic fever

10 Ocular infections due to streptococci include

    A purulent conjunctivitis
    B dacryocystitis
    C endophthalmitis
    D hordeolum
    E ulcerative keratitis

11 The gram-negative cocci *Neisseria*

    A species are aerobic or facultative anaerobic organisms
    B *gonorrhoeae* ferments glucose only
    C species grow best in cooled blood agar
    D species are oxidase positive
    E species produce exotoxins

12 *Neisseria meningitidis*

    A is prevented from causing meningococcal disease in most adults by the presence of protective serum antibodies
    B is found in the nasopharynx of asymptomatic carriers
    C type C is associated with major epidemics
    D is found in pairs in lymphocytes
    E is capsulated

13 Mycobacteria

    A are non-motile, non-capsulated, non-sporing obligate aerobes
    B induce a type IV hypersensitivity reaction
    C are known as acid and alcohol fast bacilli due to their inability to take up Gram stain
    D cause orbital cellulitis
    E cause ulcerative keratitis
    F are easily destroyed by drying

14 Which of the following features are essential for histological diagnosis of tuberculosis caused by *M. tuberculosis*?

    A Caseation
    B Epithelioid cells
    C Acid-fast bacilli

D Langhan's giant cells
E Lymphocytes

15 *M. tuberculosis*: Hypersensitivity in tuberculosis

    A crosses the placental barrier
    B results in spread
    C is associated with erythema nodosum
    D results in enhanced caseating necrosis
    E is enhanced by neonatal thymectomy

16 Which of the following statements about *Mycobacterium tuberculosis* are true?

    A *M. tuberculosis* is never a commensal in humans.
    B Past infection results in a positive Mantoux test within 48 h.
    C BCG vaccine protects 80% of those vaccinated for life.
    D *M. tuberculosis* is associated with Assman foci.
    E Miliary TB is associated with a negative Mantoux test.
    F Mantoux test is mediated by antibodies.
    G Primary sites of TB infection are lung, skin, tonsils and small intestine.

17 Which of the following are intracellular organisms?

    A *Mycobacteria*
    B *Listeria*
    C *Brucella*
    D *Toxoplasma*
    E *Salmonella*
    F *Chlamydia*
    G *Leishmania*
    H *Rickettsia*
    I *Neisseria*
    J *Nocardia asteroides*
    K *Legionella pneumophila*

18 Which of the following statements about gram-positive bacilli are true?

    A *Clostridium perfringens* is a non-motile, anaerobic, spore-forming rod.
    B Spores do not contain mRNA.
    C *Clostridium perfringens* is a commensal of the intestine.

D *Clostridium perfringens* is sensitive to penicillin.

E *Clostridium tetani* can be isolated from cerebrospinal fluid in tetanus.

19 Regarding *Bacillus* spp., which of the following are true?

A *Bacillus anthracis* is a motile aerobic spore-forming rod.

B *Bacillus cereus* is associated with panophthalmitis.

C Polymyxin is an antibiotic produced by an aerobic spore-forming bacillus.

D *Bacillus subtilis* is gram negative.

E Some spore-forming bacilli produce endotoxins.

20 With regard to corynebacteria and actinomycete group organisms,

A *Corynebacterium diphtheriae* is a capsulated, motile, gram-positive aerobe

B actinomyces are obligate anaerobes or microaerophilic bacteria that are commensals of the throat and mouth

C *Actinomyces israeli* produces sulphur granules in tissues

D *Actinomyces israeli* is implicated as a common cause of canaliculitis

E *Nocardia asteroides* is an aerobic, motile, acid-fast bacillus found in soil

21 Which of the following bacteria produce hyaluronidase?

A *Proteus*

B *Clostridium perfringens*

C *Escherichia coli*

D *Streptococcus*

E *Neisseria*

F *Staph. aureus*

22 How many of the following statements about Enterobacteriaceae are true?

A Enterobacteriaceae are bile-soluble, gram-negative, oxidase-negative bacilli.

B *E. coli* is usually a motile, lactose-fermenting, gram-negative bacillus with no urease activity.

C *Salmonella typhi* is found in the liver of typhoid carriers.

D Diagnosis of typhoid in the second week of illness is by faeces.

E *Salmonella* species are identified by agglutination tests.

23 Which of the following statements about other gram-negative bacilli are true?

A *Pseudomonas aeruginosa* is a motile, oxidase-positive, gram-negative bacillus.
B *Pseudomonas aeruginosa* produces a green pigment and antibacterial substance.
C *Pseudomonas* produces potent endotoxins responsible for its pathogenicity.
D *Haemophilus* is a gram-negative bacillus that shows 'satellitism' around strep-
   tococci in mixed culture on blood agar.
E *Haemophilus influenzae* is a normal commensal of the mouth and pharynx.

24 Live attenuated vaccines are used in the prophylaxis of

A poliomyelitis
B rubella
C hepatitis A
D measles
E smallpox
F influenza
G tuberculosis
H yellow fever
I shigella

25 *Chlamydia*

A types E–K are associated with trachoma
B is associated with Reiter's disease
C is an intracellular parasite associated with cytoplasmic inclusion bodies
D does not possess a cell wall
E type G is associated with lymphogranuloma venereum
F possesses both RNA and DNA
G is resistant to lysosomal enzymes
H possesses outer cell walls similar to gram-negative bacteria

26 Exotoxins

A are mostly enzyme lipopolysaccharides
B are heat stable
C form toxoids with ethanol
D do not usually elicit a strong antigenic response
E are produced by *Aspergillus flavus*

27 Which of the following statements about herpes simplex virus are true?

A Herpes simplex type I and II can be differentiated by complement fixation anti-body tests.

B Type I infection is subclinical in 10% of those infected.

C Giemsa stain is effective in showing eosinophilic intranuclear inclusion bodies.

D Herpes simplex virus is a double-stranded DNA virus with a helical capsid of 100 nm in diameter.

E Type II infection is associated with meningitis.

28 Varicella zoster virus

A is spread by direct contact and faeco-orally

B is associated with Lipschütz bodies

C can affect both motor and sensory nerves

D shingles may be acquired as a primary infection through vesicle contact or air-borne transmission

E complement fixation testing shows rising antibody titres in the early stages of shingles

29 Which of the following statements about cytomegalovirus are true?

A Cytomegalovirus is associated with 'owl's eye' inclusion bodies.

B IgM titres indicate active infection.

C Primary infection in pregnancy is incompatible with foetal life.

D Live attenuated vaccine is available for the immunocompromised.

E Cytomegalovirus is present in the cervix of up to 10% of healthy women.

F Cytomegalovirus is infective for animals.

30 Measles

A is caused by a paramyxovirus

B live vaccine may be transmitted

C infection is commonly associated with a secondary bacterial pneumonia

D incubation is 5–7 days

E active disease results in raised levels of IgM antibody

F infection is usually subclinical

31 Epstein–Barr virus

    A is associated with nasopharyngeal carcinoma and Burkitt's lymphoma
    B is a double-stranded RNA virus
    C specific antibodies in active disease are directed against the capsid
    D past infection is indicated by antibodies to nuclear antigens
    E is transmitted by the mosquito

32 Rubella

    A infection is associated with suboccipital lymphadenopathy
    B primary infection in pregnancy is associated with congenital cataracts
    C is a DNA togavirus easily killed by heat and UV light
    D incubation period is 7 days
    E maximum infectivity is during the time the rash is present

33 Adenovirus

    A is an RNA virus
    B has more than 40 different serotypes
    C infection is associated with a neutrophil followed by a mononuclear cell response
    D is associated with pharyngitis and latent tonsillar infection
    E is heat resistant

34 Hepatitis A

    A infection is often subclinical
    B virus can be seen in stool during clinical illness
    C is a 28 nm DNA virus
    D past infection is indicated by IgG antibody titres
    E infection can result in chronic hepatitis
    F is associated with carrier status
    G is associated with an increased risk of developing hepatoma

35 Hepatitis B

    A virus disappears from the blood with the onset of jaundice
    B vaccine consists of core antigen
    C virus can be cultured from serum
    D 'e' antigen is initially present in all cases of acute hepatitis B
    E is a DNA virus

F is associated with a T cell-mediated immune response
G causes a subclinical infection with full recovery in 65% of those infected

36 Hepatitis C

A is a single-stranded RNA virus
B is associated with post-transfusion hepatitis
C is not associated with hepatoma
D causes chronic hepatitis in 50% of those infected
E is diagnosed by serology
F incubation is up to five months

37 Human immunodeficiency virus (HIV)

A is a lentivirus
B is a double-stranded RNA retrovirus
C binds to $CD4^+$ cells via the gp41 envelope protein
D contains the enzymes protease and integrase
E results in apoptosis of T helper cells
F results in increased levels of interleukin 2
G can be isolated from blood
H infection is associated with hypergammaglobulinaemia

38 Ocular complications of HIV include

A CMV retinitis
B increased risk of intraocular lymphoma
C increased risk of herpes zoster ophthalmicus
D increased risk of cryptococcus choroiditis
E conjunctival Kaposi's sarcoma

39 *Aspergillus*

A is a yeast
B produces heat- and chemical-resistant spores
C may be found in TB lung cavities
D is associated with a type I hypersensitivity reaction
E is found routinely in 15% of persons with chronic lung disease
F is associated with eosinophilia

40 *Candida*

    A is a mucocutaneous yeast
    B grows on blood agar
    C infection resulting in vaginal candidosis is associated with the oral contraceptive pill
    D is unicellular and grows by budding
    E is the commonest cause of fungal endophthalmitis

41 The protozoan: *Acanthamoeba*

    A is found in mains water supply
    B forms pH-, chemical- and temperature-resistant cysts
    C is sensitive to chlorhexidine
    D causes uveitis
    E is a parasitic amoeba

42 Surgical gloves can be sterilised by

    A dry heat at 130°C
    B gamma radiation
    C UV radiation
    D chlorhexidine
    E steam at 130°C

43 Osteomyelitis is caused by

    A *Brucella abortus*
    B *Bordetella pertussis*
    C amyloid
    D *Staphylococcus aureus*
    E *Salmonella typhi*

MICROBIOLOGY
Answers

1 A = True   **B** = True   **C** = True   **D** = True   **E** = True

All of the organisms listed have been isolated as normal flora of the skin of the eyelids and conjunctiva.

2 A = True   **B** = True   **C** = True   **D** = True   **E** = True

See notes on Microbiology Question 5.

3 A = False   **B** = False   **C** = True   **D** = True   **E** = True

See notes on Microbiology Question 5.

4 A = False   **B** = True   **C** = True   **D** = True   **E** = True

See notes on Microbiology Question 5.

5 A = True   **B** = True   **C** = True   **D** = True   **E** = True

Staphylococci are gram-positive aerobic or facultatively anaerobic bacteria found in grape-like clusters. They are catalase positive and so cause hydrogen peroxide (H_2O_2) to bubble when in contact on a slide. The coagulase test where fibrinogen is coagulated to fibrin differentiates *Staph. aureus* (coagulase positive) from coagulase-negative staphylococci, including *Staph. epidermidis* (novobiocin sensitive), *Staph. saprophyticus* (novobiocin resistant). Staphylococci do not require special media to be cultured.

Staph. aureus is a nasal and skin commensal and is usually spread directly or indirectly (by hospital staff). Spread by air can occur due to some survival against immediate drying. Strains can be characterized by bacteriophage-typing. *Staph. aureus* produces many toxins, including:

- protein A (antiphagocytic complement-inhibiting protein that binds the Fc portion of IgG),
- haemolysins α, β and γ,
- leucocidin, an antipolymorph toxin,

- enterotoxins, heat-stable and enzyme-stable proteins that resist 30 min of boiling as well as the action of gut enzymes, produced mainly by bacteriophage group III strains when grown in carbohydrate and protein foods such as rice, act on vomiting centre of brain to induce vomiting 'staphylococcal food poisoning',
- coagulase, a fibrin-depositing enzyme inhibiting leukocyte migration and causing localization,
- hyaluronidase, an enzyme that breaks down hyaluronic acid and allows it to spread through connective tissue,
- epidermolytic toxins A and B epidermis-splitting and blister-forming toxins that cause 'scalded skin' – Ritter–Lyell's disease, and
- TSS Toxin I, which causes 'toxic shock syndrome', a multiorgan disease and state of acute shock due to septicaemia. The commonest cause is a retained foreign body such as an infected tampon or IUCD.

Infections due to *Staphylococcus aureus* include abscess, impetigo, paronychia, wound infection, osteomyelitis, endocarditis (usually right heart especially in intravenous drug abusers), septicaemia, pyaemia, pneumonia (usually secondary to influenza), food poisoning and specific toxin-related diseases (see above).

6 **A** = False   **B** = True   **C** = False   **D** = False   **E** = True

See notes on Microbiology Question 10.

7 **A** = False   **B** = False   **C** = True   **D** = True   **E** = False

See notes on Microbiology Question 10.

8 **A** = True   **B** = False   **C** = True   **D** = True   **E** = True

See notes on Microbiology Question 10.

9 **A** = False   **B** = False   **C** = True   **D** = False   **E** = False

See notes on Microbiology Question 10.

10 **A** = True   **B** = True   **C** = True   **D** = False   **E** = True

Streptococci are gram-positive cocci, catalase negative (staphylococci are catalase positive), mainly facultative anaerobes or aerobes, and prefer to grow on blood agar (or other enriched media). Many are commensals as well as pathogens. Classification is based on their appearance on blood agar.

β-Haemolytic streptococci produce a soluble haemolysin that leaves a clear zone after complete lysis of media blood cells. Further serological subdivision of β-haemolytic streptococci is by the Lancefield classification (A, B, C, D, etc.) based on the cell wall polysaccharide antigens. β-Haemolytic streptococci can also be subdivided by their *in vitro* sensitivity to bacitracin. *Strept. pyogenes* (Lancefield group A) is sensitive to bacitracin whereas Lancefield group B (gut and vaginal commensal, causes infection in new-born including septicaemia and meningitis), groups C and D (wound infections and sore throats) are resistant to bacitracin.

β-Haemolytic streptococci including *Strept. pneumoniae* (optochin sensitive) and *Strept. viridans* (optochin resistant) produce a zone of partial haemolysis around each colony (they do not possess haemolysin) with a green zone around each colony due to reduction of haemoglobin.

Strept. pyogenes is a β-haemolytic Lancefield group A streptococcus that can be further subtyped by Griffiths typing (M, R, T) based on the surface antigen M protein indicating virulence. It is a commensal of the throat in up to 25% of the population and of the nose in up to 4% of the population. Toxins produced include streptokinase, streptolysin O (oxygen-labile haemolysin) and streptolysin S (oxygen stable), hyaluronidase, erythrogenic toxin (scarlet fever – Dick test – toxin antibodies diagnostic for immunity), DNAase and leucocidin.

An allergic response to *Strept. pyogenes* infection can result in rheumatic fever or glomerulonephritis.

Strept. viridans is a β-haemolytic commensal of the mouth. It produces a green zone of haemolysis around colonies on blood agar. It is associated with subacute bacterial endocarditis on damaged heart valves only when introduced into the blood.

Strept. pneumoniae (pneumococcus) is a β-haemolytic gram-positive diplococcus. Sensitivity to optochin is an important feature as 24 h cultures do not easily differentiate it from other β-haemolytic streptococci. It is lysed by bile and is described as being bile soluble. It is encapsulated with up to 84 different antigenic types including C substance and M antigen. The pneumococcus is found in the upper respiratory tract as a commensal of the pharynx. Infections include bronchopneumonia and lobar pneumonia, sinusitus, otitis media and meningitis.

11 **A** = False   **B** = True   **C** = False   **D** = True   **E** = False

See notes on Microbiology Question 12.

12 **A** = True   **B** = True   **C** = False   **D** = False   **E** = True

Neisseria meningitidis and *Neisseria gonorrhoeae* are gram-negative strict aerobic cocci found in pairs in polymorphs (not lymphocytes). They are oxidase positive and ferment carbohydrates. *Neisseria gonorrhoeae* ferments glucose only and *Neisseria*

meningitidis ferments both glucose and maltose. Neither of them ferment sucrose. They grow best on chocolate agar (heated blood agar) with increased carbon dioxide levels.

Neisseriae are capsulated and do not produce exotoxins, but have outer pili and membrane proteins such as proteases that allow attachment and breakdown of anti-bodies such as IgA to allow invasion as well as an endotoxin effect due to lipopoly-saccharide. This endotoxin effect is a major factor of virulence.

Neisseria meningitidis is a parasite of the nasopharynx in asymptomatic carriers. It further invades in susceptible children or young adults into the blood and possibly the meninges and CSF. Serum antibodies in most adults are protective in preventing septicaemia and meningitis. Serotyping has shown type A to be associated with major epidemics and B and C to be sporadic cases.

Neisseria gonorrhoeae is responsible for gonorrhoeal ophthalmia neonatorum. Diag-nosis is established by microscopy and cultures. Thayer–Martin medium inhibits over-growth of unwanted organisms and so is more useful in isolating *Neisseria gonorrhoeae* from genitourinary samples rather than ocular culture samples. Topical erythromycin or silver nitrate is effective as treatment, as are systemic antibiotics such as erythromycin, penicillins or third-generation cephalosporins.

13 **A** = True **B** = True **C** = False **D** = True **E** = True **F** = True **G** = False

Mycobacteria are non-motile, non-sporing, non-capsulated obligate aerobic bacilli. They have a waxy cell wall that does not take up Gram stain. They are known as acid-fast bacilli (AFB) or, more accurately, acid- and alcohol-fast bacilli (AAFB) because after staining with hot, strong, carbol fuchsin the stain is retained despite attempts to remove it with a mixture of mineral acid and alcohol (Ziehl–Neelsen stain, ZN).

They have very slow generation times and require enriched media. *M. tuberculosis* grows on Lowenstein–Jensen medium. Atypical mycobacteria such as *M. fortuitum* grow on blood agar. *M. leprae* as yet cannot be cultured on artificial media.

They are resistant to drying and can survive for weeks in dust. Mycobacteria induce a slowly progressive chronic type IV granulomatous hypersensitivity reaction.

Ocular manifestations of mycobacteria infection include phlyctenular keratitis (*M. tuberculosis*), interstitial keratitis, ulcerative keratitis, orbital cellulitis and the ocular features of leprosy (Hansen's disease–*M. leprae*) such as conjunctivitis, episcleritis, corneal anaesthesia, keratitis, scleritis and iritis (the commonest cause of blindness due to leprosy).

14 **A** = False **B** = False **C** = True **D** = False **E** = False

Although the above five are features of tuberculosis, only the presence of acid-fast bacilli is essential for the diagnosis.

15 **A** = False **B** = False **C** = True **D** = True **E** = False

Hypersensitivity to TB is a type IV granulomatous reaction. Cell-mediated immunity does not cross the placental barrier. The reaction results in an aggressive immune response, inhibiting spread of the organism and resulting in greater caseating necrosis, perhaps accompanied by constitutional symptoms. Erythema nodosum is a skin manifestation of TB hypersensitivity. Neonatal thymectomy reduces the body's ability to mount a strong T cell-mediated immune response.

16 **A** = True **B** = False **C** = False **D** = True **E** = True **F** = False **G** = False

M. tuberculosis is never a commensal in humans. It is an intracellular infection. It is phagocytosed in macrophages and resists destruction by intracellular enzymes. It is thus protected from circulating antibodies and is controlled by T cell-mediated immunity. Infection can be acquired by inhalation, ingestion and inoculation. Primary sites of infection include lung, tonsils and skin.

Primary infection of pulmonary tuberculosis (childhood type) begins either in the basal segment of the upper lobe or in the apical segment of the lower lobe as a Ghon's focus. Once macrophage migration causes hilar lymph node enlargement, the resultant combination is called a Ghon's complex. These usually heal with dystrophic calcification, but may spread via bronchi (open TB, haemoptysis) or haematogenously, resulting in multiple granulomatous foci (miliary tuberculosis). This is usually found in immunosuppressed patients with a reduced hypersensitivity response.

Pulmonary tuberculosis in adults usually affects the upper lobe subapical segment, referred to as an Assmann's focus. This may heal with scarring or cavitate involving either the bronchus (broncopneumonia, open TB, haemoptysis) or pleura (pleural effusions).

TB spread may reach the Peyer's patches of the small intestine through swallowing of coughed material (intestinal obstruction).

The bacille Calmette-Guérin (BCG) vaccine is a live attenuated vaccine and protects 80% of those vaccinated for 10 years.

Immunodiagnosis is based on injecting a purified protein derivative intradermally in order to elicit a cell-mediated hypersensitivity response between 48 and 72 h. (Mantoux = syringe and needle, Heaf = spring-loaded six-needle gun). A positive Mantoux test indicates past infection either by *M. tuberculosis* or a live attenuated BCG vaccine.

Miliary TB is usually seen in the immunosuppressed and is thus associated with a negative Mantoux test.

17 **A** = True **B** = True **C** = True **D** = True **E** = True **F** = True **G** = True
   H = True **I** = True **J** = True **K** = True

The organisms listed are engulfed by macrophages or neutrophils and remain intracellular, resisting destruction by intracellular enzymes.

18 **A** = True   **B** = True   **C** = True   **D** = True   **E** = False

Clostidia are spore-forming, anaerobic, gram-positive rods. Spores are formed to allow a dormant existence in suboptimal conditions. Spores consist of a cysteine-rich kera-tin-like cortex, some cytoplasm, double-stranded DNA, ribosomes and tRNA but no mRNA. They are resistant to heat, chemicals and drying and do not reproduce or have any metabolism. They are produced by *Clostridium* and *Bacillus* species. Clostridia are mostly soil saprophytes. *Clostridium perfringens* is a non-motile anaerobic spore-forming rod and a commensal of the intestine. There are six types (A–F) depending on exotoxins produced. Type A is associated with gas gangrene and produces β-toxin (lecithinase) as well as collagenase, hyaluronidase, and deoxyribonuclease.

Clostridium perfringens is sensitive to penicillin. Treatment of gas gangrene includes surgical debridement, hyperbaric oxygen, penicillin and antitoxin against β-toxin.

Clostrium tetani is motile. Infection is usually by the spherical terminal 'drumstick' spores. It is usually present in animal intestines as well as soil and dust. It produces exotoxins that act on the CNS causing tonic spasm of voluntary muscles, eventually progressing to respiratory failure.

19 **A** = False   **B** = True   **C** = True   **D** = False   **E** = False

Bacillus species are gram-positive, aerobic, spore-forming rods. *Bacillus anthracis* is non-motile, grows on blood agar, is transmitted from animals and is responsible for anthrax due to exotoxin effects on the skin, lungs and intestines.

Bacillus cereus and *Bacillus subtilis* are associated with penetrating trauma, endophthalmitis and keratitis as well as food poisoning by their production of a poten-tially lethal exotoxin.

Antibiotics such polymyxin and bacitracin are produced by *Bacillus* species.

Endotoxins are the lipopolysaccharide constituents of gram-negative bacteria cell walls and are released on bacterial death. Spore-forming bacilli are gram positive.

20 **A** = False   **B** = True   **C** = True   **D** = True   **E** = False

Corynebacterium diphtheriae is a non-sporing, non-capsulated, non-motile, aerobic, gram-pcsitive bacillus. *Actinomyces israeli* is a gram-positive bacillus. It is an obligate anaerobe that has branched filaments and gives the appearance of sulphur granules. It is an oral and throat commensal and may cause infection of the lacrimal canaliculi (canaliculitis) and often the conjunctiva (conjunctivitis) as well as causing lung abscesses, ileitis and pelvic inflammatory disease associated with long-term use of the IUCD.

Nocardia asteroides is a motile, aerobic, filamentous, gram-positive bacillus found in soil. It is an intracellular parasite. Although a few filaments may show acid fast proper-ties, it is not acid-fast. It is responsible for granulomatous lung and skin infections, often with cerebral involvement in the immunosuppressed.

21 **A** = False **B** = True **C** = True **D** = True **E** = False **F** = True

Not all *Streptococcus* species produce hyaluronidase.

22 **A** = False **B** = True **C** = False **D** = True **E** = True

See notes on Microbiology Question 23.

23 **A** = True **B** = True **C** = False **D** = False **E** = True

Enterobacteriaceae are bile-tolerant, gram-negative, oxidase-negative bacilli. *E. coli* is a motile, lactose-fermenting, gram-negative bacillus with no urease activity. It is a commensal of the gut (except for the enteropathic enterotoxin-producing strains). It may cause infantile gastroenteritis, travellers' diarrhoea, haemorrhagic colitis and hae-molytic uraemic syndrome. It may cause sepsis of the urinary tract, wounds, perito-neum (peritonitis and septicaemia), biliary tract and is a cause of neonatal meningitis.

Salmonella are motile, non-lactose-fermenting, urease-negative, enteric pathogens causing gastroenteritis and enteric fever. Over 1000 species possess different surface antigens that are serologically identified by agglutination tests. Most species cause gastroenteritis. Four species (*S. typhi* and *S. paratyphi* A, B and C) cause enteric fever. The bacteria is transmitted by water or food and invades the gut lymphoid tissue before multiplying in macrophages and causing a second bacteraemia. They then reinfect the gut via the biliary system. Five per cent of patients with typhoid become chronic carriers with *S. typhi* colonizing the gall bladder. This may be eradicated by ciproflox-acin. The incubation period is for 1–2 weeks before headache, fever, malaise and constipation start, followed by gastrointestinal upset. Diagnosis in the first week of illness is by blood culture, in the second week by culture of the faeces, and in the third week by urine or later by serology (Widal's test) which may not be positive for at least three weeks.

Pseudomonas aeruginosa (not a member of the Enterobacteriaceae) is a strictly aerobic, flagellated, motile, oxidase-positive, gram-negative bacillus that produces green pigment. It is an opportunistic organism in the immunosuppressed. It is known to contaminate antibiotic and disinfectant solutions and is thermophilic. It produces pyocins which are themselves antibacterial as well as being useful in subtyping the organism.

Haemophilus is a gram-negative bacillus that shows satellitism around staphylococci in mixed culture on blood agar. It is a normal commensal of the mouth and pharynx.

24 **A** = True   **B** = True   **C** = False   **D** = True   **E** = True   **F** = False   **G** = True
    H = True   **I** = True

Except for hepatitis A, whose prophylactic vaccination involves a killed preparation, all
the above require live attenuated strain vaccines for prophylaxis.
    BCG (bacille Calmette-Guérin) is the vaccine for tuberculosis.

25 **A** = False   **B** = True   **C** = True   **D** = False   **E** = False   **F** = True   **G** = True
    H = True

Chlamydia are intracellular organisms. They possess a bacterial cell wall similar to
gram-negative bacteria as well as DNA, RNA, ribosomes and metabolic enzymes.
They are resistant to lysosomal enzymes. In epithelial (not inflamed) cells, large basophilic cytoplasmic inclusion bodies are also seen. (Giemsa – cytoplasmic inclusion
bodies, Papanicolaou – nuclear inclusion bodies.) Chlamydia may be serologically
subtyped. Types A–C are associated with trachoma, types D–K with sexually transmitted inclusion conjunctivitis and type L with lymphogranuloma venereum. *Chlamydia
trachomatis* is associated with non-specific urethritis and Reiter's disease (urethritis,
conjunctivitis and arthritis).

26 **A** = False   **B** = False   **C** = False   **D** = False   **E** = True

Exotoxins are usually enzymatic proteins produced mainly by gram-positive bacteria as
well as a few gram-negative (*V. cholerae, E. coli*). They are produced whilst the bacteria
are living as opposed to endotoxins (from Gram negative organisms) which are released
on bacterial death. Exotoxins are potent, strongly antigenic, usually heat-labile proteins
that form toxoids with formaldehyde and have a specific action.
    Aspergillus flavus is a fungus that infects groundnuts and produces a toxin known as
aflatoxin.

27 **A** = False   **B** = False   **C** = False   **D** = False   **E** = True

Herpes simplex, varicella zoster, cytomegalo and Epstein–Barr viruses are double-
stranded DNA viruses with icosahedral capsids of 100 nm and complete enveloped
particle of 150 nm in diameter. The particles form in cell nuclei and are able to remain
latent in the body for life.
    Type I and II herpes simplex virus can be differentiated with monoclonal antibodies by
fluorescent antibody staining of scrapings taken from skin, cornea or conjunctiva.
Complement fixation antibody testing is only useful if differentiating primary from
recurrent herpes infection. Serial blood samples show a rise in antibody titre in primary
infection and little change during recurrent infection.
    Type I is usually subclinical but in 10% may cause gingivostomatitis.

HSV is associated with Lipschütz bodies. These are epithelial cell eosinophilic intra-nuclear inclusion bodies. Papanicolaou staining demonstrates these well (Papanicolaou – nuclear inclusion bodies, Giemsa – cytoplasmic inclusion bodies).

Type II primary infection is usually sexually transmitted and may be associated with a mild meningitis.

28 **A** = False **B** = True **C** = True **D** = False **E** = True

Varicella zoster virus (a herpes virus) is a double-stranded DNA virus associated with eosinophilic nuclear inclusion bodies (Lipschütz bodies). It produces two diseases. Varicella, the primary infection, known as chickenpox, and herpes zoster, known as shingles. Patients with either are infective and the virus may be spread by direct contact with virus-filled skin vesicles or via the respiratory route through the mucosa of the upper respiratory tract. Varicella zoster virus can affect sensory ganglia, causing shingles, or affect motor nerves such as the facial nerve, causing Bell's palsy. Shingles is never acquired as a primary infection. Complement fixation is useful in showing rising antibody titres in the early stages of both varicella and zoster. Levels change very little during reactivation of zoster.

29 **A** = True **B** = True **C** = False **D** = False **E** = True **F** = False

Cytomegalovirus (a herpes virus) infection is usually asymptomatic in children. Over 50% of the UK population are thought to be seropositive. Human CMV does not infect animals. The virus remains latent, possibly in lymphocytes or macrophages, and may be reactivated. Foetal infection may be due to maternal reactivation, in which case it is usually asymptomatic, or primary maternal infection. In the latter, infection is associated with CNS involvement ranging from deafness to motor disorders and microcephaly, as well as jaundice, hepatosplenomegaly, thrombocytopenia and haemolytic anaemia.

Primary infection in pregnancy is associated with a 33% risk of foetal infection. Of these, 10% are believed to acquire cytomegalic inclusion disease (CMID). CMID has an incidence of 100 per year in the UK, and is associated with microphthalmia, chorioretinitis and strabismus.

CMV may be shed from the genitourinary route and is a source of infection to infants during childbirth. Diagnosis is by serology with IgM indicating active infection and IgG past infection, or isolation in tissue culture identifying the characteristic nuclear 'owl's eye' inclusion bodies. CMV causes severe infection in the immunocompromised and no vaccine is available.

30 **A** = True **B** = False **C** = True **D** = False **E** = True **F** = False

Measles is a paramyxovirus that is transmitted airborne in respiratory secretions early in infection. It is characterised by a prodrome of fever, nasal discharge, pharyngitis and conjunctivitis followed by a progressively generalizing rash and Koplik's spots. Symptoms may be severe with complications such as otitis media and secondary bacterial and viral pneumonia. Postinfectious encephalitis has a 50% mortality. Subacute sclerosing panencephalitis is associated with children, especially boys who acquire measles before the age of 2 years. The illness begins insidiously 7 years postmeasles with changes in behaviour, personality, intellect and progresses to death.

The incubation period for measles is between 10 and 14 days and infection is never subclinical. The virus may be isolated as well as diagnosed by a rise in IgM antibody titres. A live attenuated vaccine is routinely given and is not transmitted.

31 **A** = True   **B** = False   **C** = True   **D** = True   **E** = False

EBV is a double-stranded DNA virus belonging to the herpes group of viruses. It usually causes asymptomatic primary infection in children. However, infection in adolescence and adulthood causes infectious mononucleosis (glandular fever).

Diagnosis of active disease is by detection of circulating heterophile antibodies (Paul–Bunnell test) or by detection of antibodies against the capsid. IgM and IgG are raised in active disease, however only IgG remains later in life in low levels. Past infection may be diagnosed by the presence of nuclear antibodies which appear weeks after infection and remain present for life. It is associated with nasopharyngeal carcinoma in parts of China and Burkett's lymphoma. The link between EBV and Burkett's lymphoma in Africa is thought to be due to the presence of malaria. Humans appear to be the only host.

32 **A** = True   **B** = True   **C** = False   **D** = False   **E** = True

Rubella is a fragile RNA togavirus easily killed by heat and UV light. It is spread by droplets via the respirary tract and has an incubation period of between 14 and 21 days, averaging 18 days. Its importance lies in the risk of congenital abnormalities in children whose mothers were infected early in pregnancy. Infection is associated with mild fever, headache, general malaise and cervical, suboccipital and postauricular lymphadenopathy. A fine maculopapular rash begins over the face, spreading over the arms and trunk lasting 2 days and coincides with maximum infectivity. Primary infection early in pregnancy is associated with congenital heart disease, mental retardation and deafness. Ocular defects include cataract, microphthalmos and glaucoma.

33 **A** = False   **B** = True   **C** = True   **D** = True   **E** = False

Adenoviruses are heat-sensitive DNA viruses with more than 40 different antigenic serotypes, some of which are associated with infections of the eye. As well as serology they can be identified by isolation and immunofluorescent microscopy. Response to infection is polymorphonuclear initially followed by a mononuclear macrophage response. It is associated with pharyngitis, cough, pyrexia, latent tonsillar infection in children and ocular infections including follicular conjunctivitis.

34 A = True **B** = False **C** = False **D** = True **E** = False **F** = False **G** = False

Hepatitis A is a 28 nm RNA virus spread faeco-orally and causes nausea, vomiting, jaundice (that lasts for weeks), dark urine and pale faeces. Incubation is up to 6 weeks. Although virus isolation is not routine, it may be seen by electron microcroscopy in stool during incubation. The virus disappears with the onset of symptoms. Diagnosis is by serology. IgM indicates recent infection and IgG past infection. The virus causes acute hepatitis and is not associated with chronic hepatitis or carrier state. It is not associated with an increased risk of primary hepatoma.

35 A = False **B** = False **C** = False **D** = True **E** = True **F** = True **G** = True

Hepatitis B is a 42 nm diameter DNA virus made up of an outer protein coat and an inner protein core containing circular DNA and DNA polymerase as well as an 'e' antigen. This is collectively known as a Dane particle.

Transmission is parenteral, vertical, sexual and by close contact. Incubation is up to five months before the onset of jaundice. At this stage the virus continues to remain in the blood for many weeks after. Diagnosis is by serology, however the virus may be isolated from blood and seen under electron microscopy. It cannot be cultured.

Pathogenesis is by a cytotoxic T cell-mediated immune response which is directed against hepatocytes expressing viral antigen. Two-thirds of those infected have a subclinical infection with only 5% becoming carriers and 95% recovering fully. Of the remaining one-third, three-quarters undergo acute hepatitis with 99% recovery and 1% developing fulminant hepatitis. The remaining one-quarter (i.e. approximately 10%) develop chronic hepatitis, one-third of whom continue with chronic persistent hepatitis and two-thirds progress to chronic active hepatitis with a risk of developing cirrhosis.

Overall mortality is 1%, with carriers and those with chronic hepatitis having an increased risk of developing primary hepatoma.

HBeAg 'e' antigen found in the inner core, if found persistently in the blood is associated with 'super' highly infectious carrier status, but, is present in all acute cases initially.

A vaccine exists against hepatitis B and consists of the surface antigen HBsAg of the virus without the core antigen or protein. It is produced by cloning the surface antigen gene in yeast.

36 A = True **B** = True **C** = False **D** = True **E** = True **F** = False

Hepatitis C is a single-stranded RNA virus between 30 and 60 nm in size. It is transmitted parenterally and associated with post-transfusion hepatitis. Screening of donated blood for hepatitis C virus is now routine in the UK. It has an incubation period of up to ten weeks and from then on may be diagnosed by serology (anti-HCV antibodies). Fifty per cent of those infected recover fully. The remaining 50% develop chronic hepatitis. Of those, 50% continue insidiously with chronic persistent hepatitis whereas the remaining 50% (25% of total) develop chronic active hepatitis. Of those patients with chronic active hepatitis, two-thirds remain with chronic active hepatitis only and one-third of patients (over 10% of total) go on to develop cirrhosis of the liver. Chronic disease is associated with an increased risk of primary hepatoma.

37 **A** = True   **B** = False   **C** = False   **D** = True   **E** = True   **F** = False   **G** = True
   H = True

HIV is a single-stranded RNA retrovirus with a lentivirus-like life cycle. It consists of a protein core encasing the genome RNA and the enzymes reverse transcriptase, integrase and protease. It is surrounded by a complex lipid envelope containing the gp120 and gp41 envelope proteins. The core contains the p24 protein. These proteins are coded for by structural genes *gag*, *pol* and *env* in the genome. Modified genes include *tat*, *rev* and *ref* genes that regulate viral activity. The virus binds to CD4$^+$ cells via its gp120 envelope protein. These cells include T helper cells, monocytes, macrophages, some B cells and microglial cells in the CNS. Following production of DNA (reverse transcriptase) the double-stranded DNA is integrated into the host-cell genome (integrase). This is followed by transcription and translation and then post-transcriptional modifications (protease) of virus proteins. The virus assembles and buds off from the host cell. Cytopathicity is by enhancing cell destruction. This may be done directly by cell-to-cell fusion, autofusion, accumulation of damaging intracellular components or apoptosis of T helper cells (terminal differentiation by programmed cell death). Indirect cell destruction occurs by clearance of gp120-coated cells by T cytotoxic cells and killer cells. HIV also decreases the production of interleukin 2 by the destruction of T helper cells. This reduces the T cell-stimulating response. HIV stimulates certain B cells to induce polyclonal immunoglobulin production, resulting in hypergammaglobulinaemia. HIV may be isolated from blood or body fluids either free or inside monocytes, macrophages or lymphocytes, however, diagnosis is based on the presence of antibodies against the virus.

38 **A** = True   **B** = True   **C** = True   **D** = True   **E** = True

Ocular complications of HIV are usually seen with the onset of the acquired immune deficiency syndrome (AIDS) and develops in about 75% of AIDS patients. They can be classified into retinal microangiopathies, opportunistic infections, tumours and neurological lesions affecting the eyes.

Cottonwool spots are a common finding in AIDS. Opportunistic infections such as CMV retinitis, herpes zoster ophthalmicus and cryptococcus choroiditis are commonly seen. Kaposi's sarcoma affects 25% of AIDS patients and may be found on the eyelids or the conjunctiva. Lymphomas of the eye have a greater incidence in AIDS.

39 A = False **B** = False **C** = True **D** = True **E** = True **F** = True

Aspergillus is a saprophytic thermophilic filamentous fungus (or mould). *Aspergillus fumigatus* is the commonest infecting species. It produces chemical- and heat-sensitive reproductive spores as well as filamentous projections (hyphae) which combine and intertwine to be described as a mycelium. Aspergillus grows on decaying leaves and plants and are found in high concentrations in the air during autumn. It can be grown routinely in 15% of asymptomatic patients with chronic lung disease. It is responsible for allergic bronchopulmonary aspergillosis where it grows on bronchial walls resulting in an allergic asthmatic type I hypersensitivity reaction accompanied by eosinophilia.

In a separate disease it may colonize damaged cystic or TB lung cavities and produce a ball of mycelium known as an aspergilloma that can be relatively asymptomatic or result in haemoptysis. It commonly results in ocular infections, the main ones being keratitis and endophthalmitis, especially postsurgery or postinjury, when resistance is reduced either due to corticosteroid therapy or immunosuppression.

40 A = True **B** = True **C** = True **D** = True **E** = True

Candida is a unicellular yeast (a eukaryote) that grows by budding and causes mucocutaneous and deep systemic infections. It is a commensal of the skin, mouth, gastrointestinal tract and genitourinary tract.

Candida albicans is the commonest cause of candidosis. It is also the commonest cause of fungal endophthalmitis and also causes keratitis. It grows well on blood agar as well as fungal media, producing large 'cottage cheese' like colonies.

The use of oral contraceptives, as well as corticosteroids, antibiotics and cytotoxic drugs can predispose to candidosis.

41 A = True **B** = True **C** = True **D** = True **E** = False

Acanthamoeba is a free-living amoeba found in soil, air, ponds and mains water. It can adopt two phases, either an active trophozoite, or a cyst which remains dormant and resistant to temperature, pH and chemical extremes. Due to its presence in mains water it can contaminate contact lenses via their storage cases. Common species include *A. castellania* and *A. polyphaga*.

Ocular infections include epithelial and stromal keratitis, uveitis and optic neuritis. Treatment is with dipropamide, polyhexamethylene biguanide, propamidine esothionate (Brolene) and neomycin, however it is sensitive to chlorhexidine.

42 **A** = False   **B** = True   **C** = False   **D** = False   **E** = True

Surgical gloves would melt if exposed to dry heat at 130°C and would only be disinfected on exposure to UV radiation or chlorhexidine.

43 **A** = True   **B** = False   **C** = False   **D** = True   **E** = True

Secondary amyloidosis often occurs secondary to chronic disease including tuberculosis, rheumatoid arthritis, leprosy, osteomyelitis and multiple myeloma.

Structured Essay Plans

Note: Each essay summary provides a suggested essay structure with key points ordered according to importance. For further details of the 'traffic light' system used to prioritise points, please refer to the Preface (p. vii).

Essay Structure 1: *Outline the Differences Between the Sympathetic and Parasympathetic Divisions of the Autonomic Nervous System*

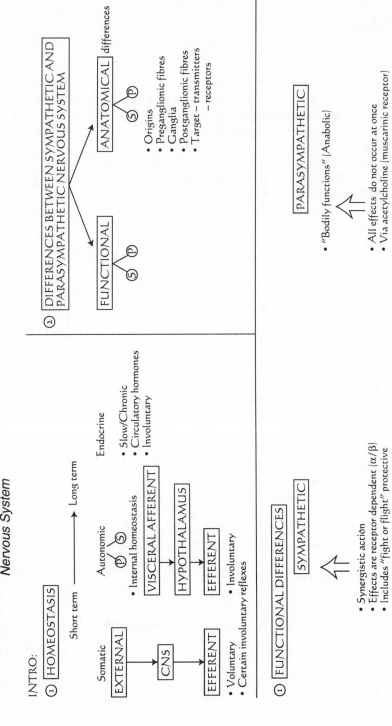

Examples (From "Head to toe"):

SYMPATHETIC

- Brain (↑alertness)
- ↑ pupil size • ↓ lens convexity • ↓ secretions
- Lungs/bronchodilation
- Heart (↑HR/SV)
- GI tract (relax smooth muscle, contract sphincters)
- Bladder (relax muscle, contract sphincter)
- Skin (vasoconstriction, sweating)
- Liver/pancreas (fat/CHO metabolism)
- Blood vessels (α/β)
- Genitals (ejaculation)

(NB: Erection/Ejaculation = "Point" (erection) and "Shoot" (ejaculation)

RECEPTORS:

- α (alpha) – usu. EXCITATORY (inhibitory in GI tract)
- β (beta) – usu. INHIBITORY (excitatory in heart)
  (β₁ – cardiac, β₂ – bronchi/blood vessels)
- Cholinergic – sweat glands
  – arteriolar smooth muscle in skeletal muscle

PARASYMPATHETIC

- ↓ pupil size • ↑ lens convexity
- ↑ secretions (tears, saliva, nasal, bronchi, gut)
- Bronchoconstriction
- Heart (↓HR)
- GI tract (contract smooth muscle, relax sphincter)
- Ureter/bladder
- Genitals (erection)

RECEPTORS:

- NICOTINIC • Autonomic ganglion cells
  • N–M junction
  • (Adrenal medulla)

- MUSCARINIC • All postganglionic parasympathetic receptors

Essay Structure 1 cont.

② ANATOMICAL DIFFERENCES

(i) SYMPATHETIC

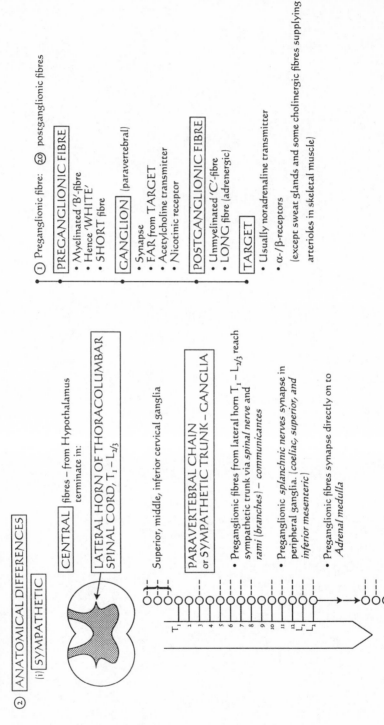

① Preganglionic fibre: •—○ ② postganglionic fibres

PREGANGLIONIC FIBRE
- Myelinated 'B'-fibre
- Hence WHITE'
- SHORT fibre

GANGLION (paravertebral)
- Synapse
- FAR from TARGET
- Acetylcholine transmitter
- Nicotinic receptor

POSTGANGLIONIC FIBRE
- Unmyelinated 'C'-fibre
- LONG fibre (adrenergic)

TARGET
- Usually noradrenaline transmitter
- α-/β-receptors
  (except sweat glands and some cholinergic fibres supplying arterioles in skeletal muscle)

CENTRAL fibres – from Hypothalamus terminate in:

LATERAL HORN OF THORACOLUMBAR SPINAL CORD, $T_1 – L_{2/3}$

Superior, middle, inferior cervical ganglia

PARAVERTEBRAL CHAIN or SYMPATHETIC TRUNK – GANGLIA

- Preganglionic fibres from lateral horn $T_1 – L_{2/3}$ reach sympathetic trunk via *spinal nerve and rami (branches) – communicantes*
- Preganglionic *splanchnic nerves synapse in peripheral ganglia. (coeliac, superior, and inferior mesenteric)*
- Preganglionic fibres synapse directly on to *Adrenal medulla*

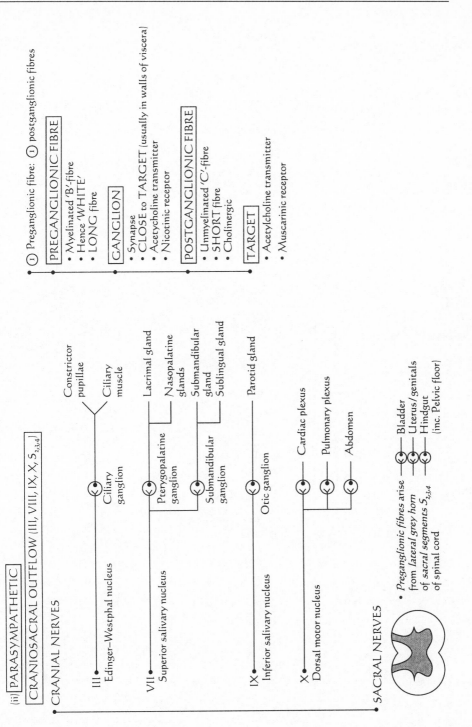

Essay Structure 2: *Describe the Mechanisms by Which Blood Flow Through a Tissue is Controlled*

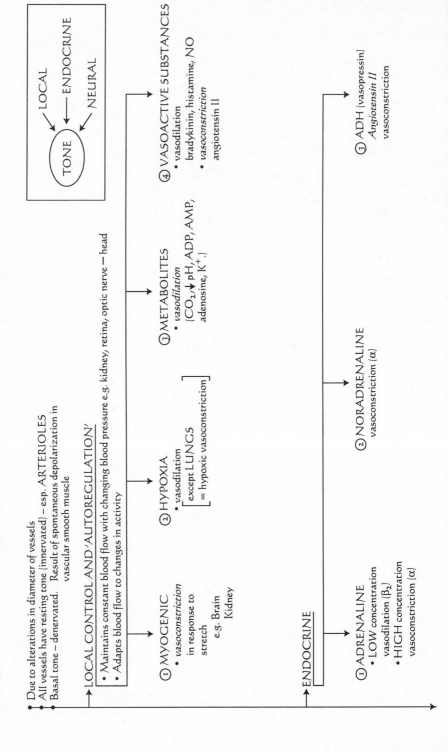

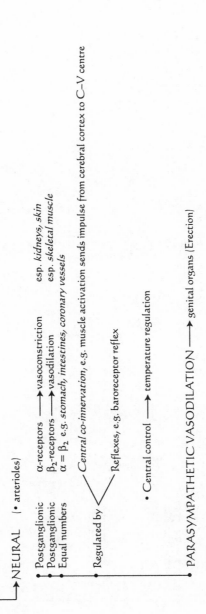

NEURAL   (• arterioles)

Postganglionic   α-receptors ⟶ vasoconstriction   esp. *kidneys, skin*
Postganglionic   β₂-receptors ⟶ vasodilation   esp. *skeletal muscle*
Equal numbers $\alpha = \beta_2$ e.g. *stomach, intestines, coronary vessels*

Central co-innervation, e.g. muscle activation sends impulse from cerebral cortex to C–V centre

Regulated by
Reflexes, e.g. baroreceptor reflex

• Central control ⟶ temperature regulation

PARASYMPATHETIC VASODILATION ⟶ genital organs (Erection)

Essay Structure 3: *Describe the Mechanism of Photopic and Scotopic Vision*

(i) MAIN OUTLINE
(ii) BACKGROUND

INTRODUCTION

BRIGHTNESS
QUALITATIVE DIFFERENCE - Between *brightness* and *darkness* perception

PHOTOPIC VISION
SCOTOPIC VISION

MECHANISMS

PHOTORECEPTOR
CONE – PHOTOPIC
ROD – SCOTOPIC

LOCAL CONTRAST PRESERVATION

ON/OFF RETINAL CHANNELS
BIPOLAR CELLS
GANGLION CELLS
LGN
VISUAL CORTEX

LATERAL INHIBITION
HORIZONTAL CELLS
AMACRINE CELLS

IMPORTANT FEATURES

PHOTORECEPTORS
CENTRE-SURROUND
ON/OFF CHANNELS

CONCLUSION

Separate mechanisms for photopic and scotopic vision
Begins at PHOTORECEPTOR level
Visual system organized to detect CONTRAST rather than absolute levels of light
ON and OFF channels
Centre-Surround
Border contrast mainly at RETINAL level
Area contrast at Retina/LGN/?CORTEX/?BEYOND

BACKGROUND

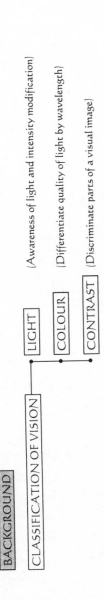

CLASSIFICATION OF VISION
- LIGHT (Awareness of light and intensity modification)
- COLOUR (Differentiate quality of light by wavelength)
- CONTRAST (Discriminate parts of a visual image)

LIGHT SENSE • INTENSITY due to • Light source • Object reflectance

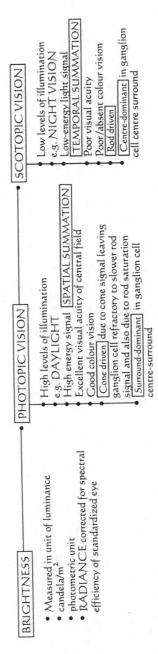

BRIGHTNESS
- Measured in unit of luminance candela/m²
- photometric unit
- RADIANCE corrected for spectral efficiency of standardized eye

PHOTOPIC VISION
- High levels of illumination e.g. DAYLIGHT
- High energy signal SPATIAL SUMMATION
- Excellent visual acuity of central field
- Good colour vision
- Cone driven due to cone signal leaving ganglion cell refractory to slower rod signal and also due to rod saturation
- Surround-dominant in ganglion cell centre-surround

SCOTOPIC VISION
- Low levels of illumination e.g. NIGHT VISION
- Low-energy light signal TEMPORAL SUMMATION
- Poor visual acuity
- Poor/absent colour vision
- Rod driven
- Centre-dominant in ganglion cell centre surround

QUALITATIVE DIFFERENCE
- Between perception of *brightness* and *darkness*
- Not just variation in intensity
- Carried by TWO DIFFERENT POPULATIONS OF CELLS. Often with opposite responses, e.g. ON and OFF cells

Essay Structure 3 cont.

• VISUAL SYSTEM ORGANIZED TO DETECT CONTRAST establishing BORDERS rather than absolute levels of light

VISUAL PATHWAY

LIGHT

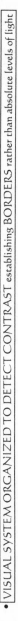
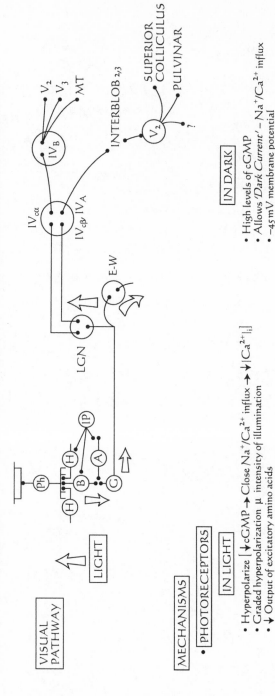

MECHANISMS

• PHOTORECEPTORS

IN LIGHT

• Hyperpolarize [$\downarrow$cGMP $\rightarrow$ Close Na^+/Ca^{2+} influx $\rightarrow$ $\downarrow|Ca^{2+}|_i$]
• Graded hyperpolarization μ intensity of illumination
• $\rightarrow$ Output of excitatory amino acids

IN DARK

• High levels of cGMP
• Allows 'Dark Current' – Na^+/Ca^{2+} influx
• –45mV membrane potential

• CONE – PHOTOPIC

4–5 million
Peak density in fovea (200 000/mm²)
Foveola is deficient in Ⓢ cones (BLUE)

RESPONSE

- High threshold with regards to background light
- Graded over 3 log units light intensity above background
- Faster response time
- ③ TYPES of photochemicals with peak absorbances at light wavelengths of 445, 535 and 570 nm Ⓢ Ⓜ Ⓛ

• RODS – SCOTOPIC

80–110 million
Peak density in a horizontal elliptical ring between nerve head and macula
(superior retina 160 000/mm²)

RESPONSE

- Lowest absolute threshold to flashes on dark background
- Graded over 3 log units light intensity above background
- Slower recovery
- Peak sensitivity at 496 nm
  Sensitive to LOW ENERGY BLUE LIGHT
  Red light requires 3 log units greater illuminance under same conditions
- Easily saturated with increased light intensity
  (Bleaching 10% of pigment causes 100-fold increase in threshold)

BEYOND PHOTORECEPTORS

NOTE:

Ⓞ Absolute levels of light

LOCAL CONTRAST PRESERVATION

Ⓞ Absolute levels of light

- Should remain constant with changes in illumination
- Based on RATIO – irrelevant of type of definition (i.e. Weber's Law, Michelson Contrast)
- e.g. ① MACH BANDS (1865) – Border contrast
- e.g.

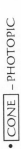

- Simultaneous contrast. Neutral object brighter or darker depending on adjacent region. ABSOLUTE ILLUMINANCE VARIABLE

Essay Structure 3 cont.

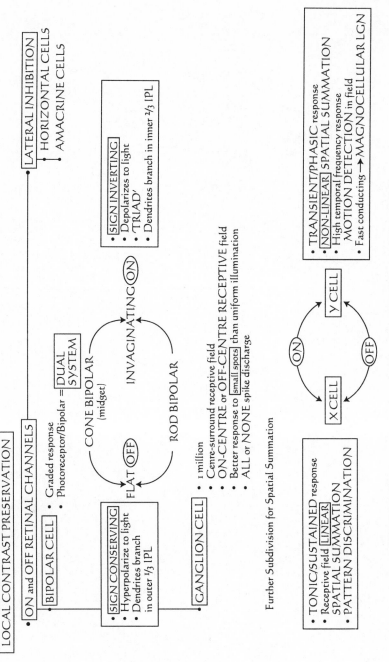

LOCAL CONTRAST PRESERVATION

ON and OFF RETINAL CHANNELS

LATERAL INHIBITION
- HORIZONTAL CELLS
- AMACRINE CELLS

BIPOLAR CELL
- Graded response
- Photoreceptor/Bipolar = DUAL SYSTEM

SIGN CONSERVING
- Hyperpolarize to light
- Dendrites branch in outer ⅓ IPL

SIGN INVERTING
- Depolarizes to light
- 'TRIAD'
- Dendrites branch in inner ⅔ IPL

CONE BIPOLAR
(midget)

FLAT (OFF)   INVAGINATING (ON)

ROD BIPOLAR

GANGLION CELL
- 1 million
- Centre-surround receptive field
- ON-CENTRE or OFF-CENTRE RECEPTIVE field
- Better response to small spots than uniform illumination
- ALL or NONE spike discharge

Further Subdivision for Spatial Summation

TONIC/SUSTAINED response
- Receptive field LINEAR
- SPATIAL SUMMATION
- PATTERN DISCRIMINATION

X CELL   Y CELL

ON   OFF

TRANSIENT/PHASIC response
- NON-LINEAR SPATIAL SUMMATION
- High temporal frequency response
- MOTION DETECTION in field
- Fast conducting → MAGNOCELLULAR LGN

- Ganglion cells from a DUAL SYSTEM of parallel regular mosaic of ON-CENTRE and OFF-CENTRE channels that sample retinal image independently
- Greater ROD CONVERGENCE than cone convergence on to ganglion cell

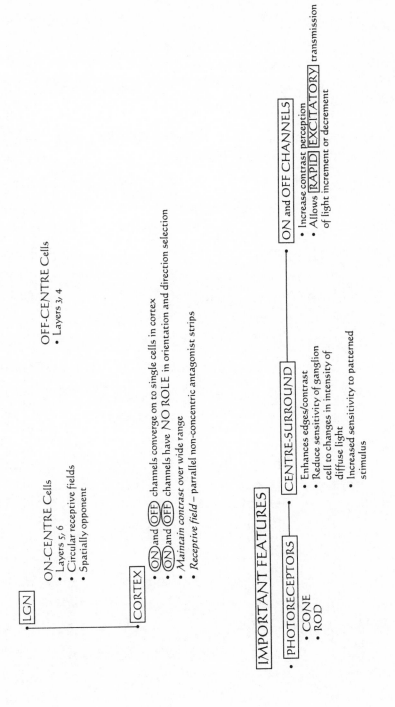

LGN

ON-CENTRE Cells
• Layers 5, 6
• Circular receptive fields
• Spatially opponent

OFF-CENTRE Cells
• Layers 3, 4

CORTEX
• (ON) and (OFF) channels converge on to single cells in cortex
• (ON) and (OFF) channels have NO ROLE in orientation and direction selection
• *Maintain contrast over wide range*
• *Receptive field – parrallel non-concentric antagonist strips*

IMPORTANT FEATURES

PHOTORECEPTORS
• CONE
• ROD

CENTRE-SURROUND
• Enhances edges/contrast
• Reduce sensitivity of ganglion cell to changes in intensity of diffuse light
• Increased sensitivity to patterned stimulus

ON and OFF CHANNELS
• Increase contrast perception
• Allows RAPID EXCITATORY transmission of light increment or decrement

Essay Structure 4: *Describe the Mechanisms Underlying the Perception of Colour*

INTRO
- COLOUR VISION → HISTORY OF COLOUR SPECTRUM → HERING'S THEORY OF COLOUR OPPONENCY

(i) MAIN OUTLINE
(ii) BACKGROUND
(iii) PARVOCELLULAR vs MAGNOCELLULAR

MECHANISMS
- COLOUR CHANNELS IN PARALLEL TO LUMINANCE CHANNELS
- LEVEL OF:

  RETINA
  - CONES • Trichomatic receptors
  - HORIZONTAL CELL • Centre-surround
  - BIPOLAR CELL • On/off pathway
  - GANGLION CELL • Colour opponency
    • Tonic/Phasic cells

  LGN
  - Parvocellular pathway

  VISUAL CORTEX
  - Foveal representation
  - Double opponency
  - Blob cells
  - V_4

CONCLUSION
- Colour perception is a parallel pathway
- RETINA
  - Trichomatic receptors → CHROMATIC PATHWAY → LGN → PARVOCELLULAR → VISUAL CORTEX → COLOUR
  - Opponency → ACHROMATIC PATHWAY (Luminance) → Magnocellular

  Activity
  Motion
  Depth

BACKGROUND

COLOUR VISION
- Sensory phenomenon
- Poorly understood mechanism
- 85% population constancy
- Related to colours of surroundings
- Combination of:
  1. light from surrounding objects
  2. light from objects
  3. state of light adaptation

HISTORY OF COLOUR SPECTRUM
Maxwell (1856), Helmholtz (1867)

TRICHOMATIC THEORY
- (3) Receptor types S M L cones
  440 535 567
- 'Hues' due to overlap of spectral sensitivity

BUT, HERING (1878) ASKED:
- YELLOW should thus be a mixture of Red/Green but instead is PRIMARY
- 'Reddish-Green' (or Bluish-Yellow) is never seen in nature.

Hence, HERING'S THEORY OF COLOUR OPPONENCY
- (4) Basic hues RED YELLOW GREEN BLUE
- PAIRED and OPPONENT processes
  - Red-Green – mutually exclusive
  - Blue-Yellow – mutually exclusive
- Achromatic dimension BLACK-WHITE opponent system – accounts for PINK, MAROON etc.
- Other colour combinations are HUES
- CONCLUSION
- (6) BASIC COLOURS coded by (3) – opponent process
RED-GREEN BLUE-YELLOW BLACK-WHITE

MECHANISMS
- Colour channels in parallel to luminance channels
- Colour channels respond to changes in wavelength and are processed independently and in parallel to changes in light intensity (luminance)

CONES
- (3) Classes
- Spectral characteristic (photopigments)
- Retinal location 1 MACULA/NASAL RETINA 2 S CONES = 2° eccentric

HORIZONTAL CELL
- Spatial organization
- RECEPTIVE FIELD Centre-surround

BIPOLAR CELL
- On/off pathways
- RECEPTIVE FIELD ON-centre/OFF-centre

Essay Structure 4 cont.

GANGLION CELL
- 1st site of COLOUR OPPONENCY
- (1+) ganglion cell types
- Receptive field – ON centres or OFF centres (excited by increment or decrement)
- 5:1 RED – GREEN : BLUE – YELLOW opponency
- ② MAJOR CLASSES OF GANGLION CELLS:

TONIC (main)	PHASIC
① Smaller ganglion cells	① Large cell bodies
② Slower conduction velocity	② Fast conduction velocity
③ Small dendritic and receptive field size	③ Large dendritic and receptive field size
④ Sustained (tonic) response	④ Short (phasic) response
⑤ Project to PARVOCELLULAR layers of LGN	⑤ Project to MAGNOCELLULAR layers of LGN
⑥ MAIN COLOUR OPPONENT PROCESSOR	⑥ MAIN PROCESSOR OF LUMINANCE CONTRAST
• Colour selective	• Colour blind
• Low-contrast sensitivity	• High-contrast sensitivity
• High resolution	• Low resolution
• Slow	• Fast

RED – GREEN OPPONENT	vs	BLUE – YELLOW OPPONENT
• Smaller receptive field size		• Larger receptive field size
• Clear spatial resolution and antagonism		• Poor spatial resolution
• Higher temporal resolution		• Lower onset latency – lower temporal resolution
• Flicker fusion frequency = 60–70 Hz		• Flicker fusion frequency = 35 Hz
		SIMILAR TO RODS

RAPID SEQUENCE STIMULI RESOLVED FASTER/EASIER

e.g. Red – Green Opponency ON-centre/OFF-surround

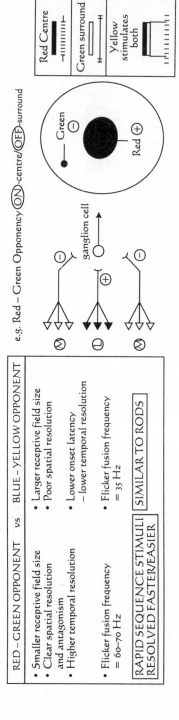

ganglion cell

Green
Red

Red Centre
Green surround
Yellow stimulates both

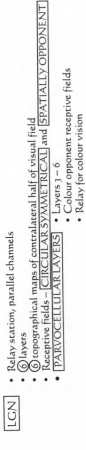

LGN
- Relay station, parallel channels
- 6 layers
- 6 topographical maps of contralateral half of visual field
- Receptive fields – CIRCULAR SYMMETRICAL and SPATIALLY OPPONENT
- PARVOCELLULAR LAYERS
  • Layers 3 – 6
  • Colour opponent receptive fields
  • Relay for colour vision

VISUAL CORTEX
- Larger representation of fovea
- Field – includes DOUBLE OPPONENCY
- Receives PARVOCELLULAR (P) and MAGNOCELLULAR (M) pathways
- No analysis of vision occurs at V_1

POSSIBLE PATHWAYS

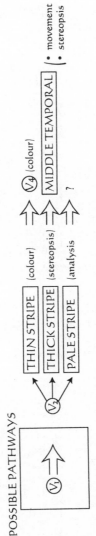

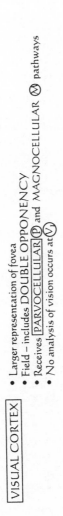

THIN STRIPE (colour)

THICK STRIPE (stereopsis)

PALE STRIPE (analysis)

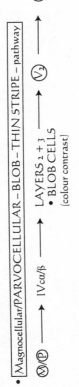

V_4 (colour)

MIDDLE TEMPORAL (• movement • stereopsis)

?

- Magnocellular/PARVOCELLULAR – BLOB – THIN STRIPE – pathway

M/P ⟶ $IVc\alpha/\beta$ ⟶ LAYERS 2 + 3
• BLOB CELLS (colour contrast) ⟶ V_2 ⟶ V_4

• COLOUR
• Low Acuity

Essay Structure 4 cont.

COMPARISON OF PARVOCELLULAR AND MAGNOCELLULAR PATHWAYS

LGN

- 6 Layers
- Relay station, parallel channels
- 6 Topographical maps of contralateral-half of visual field
- Receptive fields – CIRCULAR SYMMETRICAL and SPATIALLY OPPONENT

PARVOCELLULAR LAYER

- 4 Layers (3 – 6)
- 2 x central 20°, 2 x peripheral field
- COLOUR OPPONENT receptive fields
- Sustained response
- Small receptive field
- Receive input from slow/medium-velocity axons
- Send slow/medium-velocity signal to striate cortex
- Up to 20% lack clearcut colour sensitivity
- Receptive field 80% – COLOUR OPPONENT
  CENTRE-SURROUND

  20% – CENTRE-ONLY
  COLOUR OPPONENT
  BROADBAND

- RELAY STATION FOR COLOUR VISION
- Useful for visual activity only in the presence of
  HIGH CONTRAST

MAGNOCELLULAR LAYER

- 2 Layers (1 and 2)
- 8 – 10% of LGN volume
- Lack of colour opponency
- Transient response
- Large receptive field
- Receive input from fast velocity axons
- Send high-velocity signal to striate cortex
- High-contrast sensitivity

- RELAY STATION FOR CONTRAST VISION

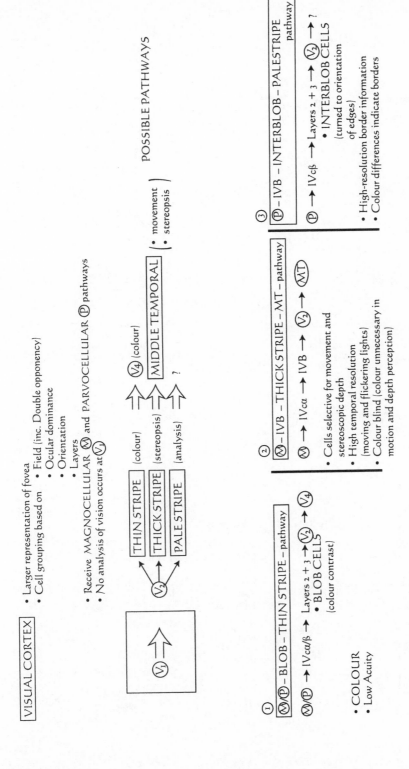

Essay Structure 5: *Describe the Supranuclear Control of Ocular Movements*

KEY FEATURES

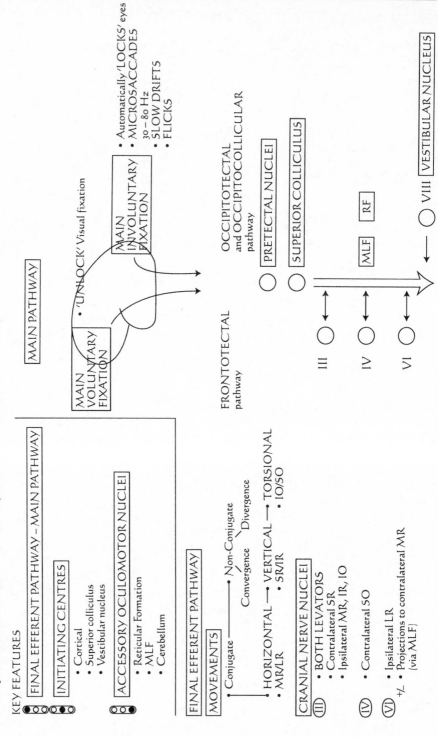

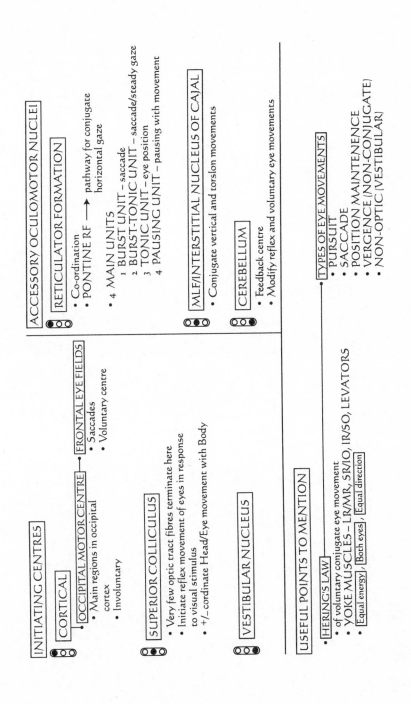

INITIATING CENTRES

CORTICAL

OCCIPITAL MOTOR CENTRE
• Main regions in occipital cortex
• Involuntary

FRONTAL EYE FIELDS
• Saccades
• Voluntary centre

SUPERIOR COLLICULUS
• Very few optic tract fibres terminate here
• Initiate reflex movement of eyes in response to visual stimulus
• +/- cordinate Head/Eye movement with Body

VESTIBULAR NUCLEUS

ACCESSORY OCULOMOTOR NUCLEI

RETICULATOR FORMATION
• Co-ordination
• PONTINE RF → pathway for conjugate horizontal gaze
• 4 MAIN UNITS
  1 BURST UNIT – saccade
  2 BURST-TONIC UNIT – saccade/steady gaze
  3 TONIC UNIT – eye position
  4 PAUSING UNIT – pausing with movement

MLF/INTERSTITIAL NUCLEUS OF CAJAL
• Conjugate vertical and torsion movements

CEREBELLUM
• Feedback centre
• Modify reflex and voluntary eye movements

TYPES OF EYE MOVEMENTS
• PURSUIT
• SACCADE
• POSITION MAINTENENCE
• VERGENCE (NON-CONJUGATE)
• NON-OPTIC (VESTIBULAR)

USEFUL POINTS TO MENTION

HERING'S LAW
• of voluntary conjugate eye movement
• YOKE MUSCLES – LR/MR, SR/IO, IR/SO, LEVATORS
• Equal energy , Both eyes , Equal direction

Essay Structure 5 cont.

RiMLF = Rostral Interstitial Nucleus of Medial Longitudinal Fasciculus

PPRF = Paramedianpontine Reticular Formation

TYPES OF EYE MOVEMENT

② SACCADIC (or RAPID EYE MVT)
- Function: Rapidly bring object of interest interest on to fovea
- Types:
  - REFIXATION e.g. Reading Eccentric target to fovea
  - VOLUNTARY e.g. Command
  - REFLEX e.g. Head movements
- Pathways initiated from:

① Frontal lobe

Midbrain Pretectal area

② *Brainstem* • Midbrain • Pons

RETICULAR FORMATION → SACCADES

③ SUPERIOR COLLICULUS
- Reflex
- Spontaneous

→ CONTRALATERAL PPRF → SACCADES

VERTICAL SACCADES | HORIZONTAL SACCADES

- LATENCY: LONG 200ms
- Velocity: FAST 30 – 700 degrees/s
- Control:
  - Sampled data
  - Pre-programmed/ballistic
  - Frontal lobe/occipitoparietal/Superior Colliculus
  - Cerebellum moderates amplitude
  - VISION SUPPRESSED DURING SACCADE

- Tests: REFIXATION ROTATION CALORICS OKN

BACKGROUND

① PURSUIT/SLOW EYE MOVEMENTS
- Function: Hold image of moving target on fovea
- Pathway:

Occipito-parietal lobe

Midbrain pretectal area

VERTICAL MVTS.
- riMLF → III, IV
- assoc. with vertical saccadic pathway

HORIZONTAL MVTS.
- PPRF (nr. VI nuc.)
- riMLF

- Stimulus: Moving target NEAR fovea
- Latency: SHORT 125 ms
- Velocity: SLOW 30 degrees/s (accurately) up to 100 degrees/s
- Control: continuous
- Tests: DOLLS HEAD ROTATION OKN

③ POSITION MAINTENANCE
- Function: Maintain eye position on a target
- Pathway:

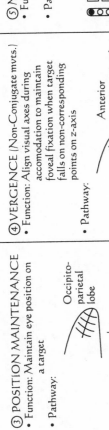

Occipito-parietal lobe → Midbrain pretectal area

VERTICAL MVTS.   HORIZONTAL MVTS.

- Stimulus: Visual interest and attention
- Velocity:
  - RAPID Flicks and microsaccades
  - SLOW Drifts

④ VERGENCE (Non-Conjugate mvts.)
- Function: Align visual axes during accomodation to maintain foveal fixation when target falls on non-corresponding points on z-axis
- Pathway:

Anterior occipitoparietal area → Midbrain/pons pretectal area

- straight to:
  III NUCLEUS
  - By-passing MLF.
  - III – interneurones – VI
- Stimulus: Retinal disparity
- Latency: 160 ms
- Velocity: < 20 degrees/s
- Control: Continuous ? unknown
- Test: DISTANT – TO – NEAR ACCOMMODATION

⑤ NON-OPTIC REFLEX (VESTIBULAR)
- Function: Maintain eye position with changes in Head and Body movement.
- Pathway:

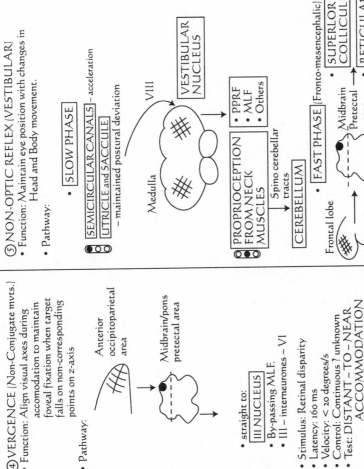

SLOW PHASE

SEMICIRCULAR CANALS – acceleration
UTRICLE and SACCULE – maintained postural deviation

VIII → Medulla → VESTIBULAR NUCLEUS

PROPRIOCEPTION FROM NECK MUSCLES
- PPRF
- MLF
- Others

Spino cerebellar tracts

CEREBELLUM

FAST PHASE (Fronto-mesencephalic)

Frontal lobe → Midbrain Pretectal area → SUPERIOR COLLICULUS → RETICULAR FORMATION

- Stimulus: Stimulation of semicircular canals, utricles and saccules
- Latency: VERY SHORT 100 ms
- Velocity: (Slow phase) up to 300 degrees/s
- Test: TAPE or DRUM.

Essay Structure 6: *Discuss the Electrophysiological Investigations of the Visual Pathway*

INTRO
- Visual system generates potentials ⟨ Spontaneously (EOG) / In response to stimulus (VEP, ERG, PERG)

- Electrical signals generated at level of ⬛EYE ⬛⬛⬛VISUAL CORTEX ⬛⬛⬛LGN

- VEP -optic N/macula. ERG -peripheral retina. PERG -central retina. EOG -RPE/Photoreceptor interaction

---

ERG
- Electroretinogram
- Recording of the summation of potential changes in the retinal layers in response to light stimulation

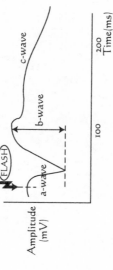

METHOD: Corneal electrodes can be contact lens or non-contact lens

- *a-wave* • PHOTORECEPTOR CELL BODY
  - Cone component/Rod component
- *b-wave* • BIPOLAR CELLS DRIVING MÜLLER CELLS.
  - Rod bipolar cell response is largest
- *c-wave* • RPE
  - Very little used

VEP • *Visual Evoked Potential*

METHOD: Electrode placed over each visual cortex
1. BLACK and WHITE checkerboard reversal
2. PATTERN ONSET - Greyscreen to checkerboard.
3. FLASH – Individual variability, useful in subjects not fixating and therefore children.
   - Consistency between hemispheres

[amplitude(μV) graph: N75, P100, N135, PATTERN VEP, Time(ms)]

- P100 Latency – most useful
  – usually constant

USE: • OPTIC NERVE DEMYELINATION e.g. MS – VEP delay
- ISCHAEMIC LESIONS – Altered wave amplitude
- COMPRESSIVE LESIONS – Delay and altered amplitude
- MACULAR DISEASE – delayed VEP

TYPES OF ERG:

① SINGLE BRIGHT WHITE LIGHT FLASH (SBLF)
- Mixed Rod/Cone response

② SCOTOPIC ERG
- Dim light (white or blue) below cone threshold
- Pure Rod response

③ 30Hz Flicker
- cone response only
- sinusoidal wave-like response

④ PHOTOPIC ERG
- Background to saturate rods
- Bright flash – cone response only

⑤ OSCILLATION RESPONSE
- Begin at 150Hz – to – 2000Hz
- Filter out a- and b- waves
- Oscillatory waves overlay on ascending limb of b-wave
- Probable HORIZONTAL CELL/AMACRINE CELL ORIGIN

USE:
- PERIPHERAL RETINA
- Generated by cells distal to ganglion cell.
- NB: DUAL CIRCULATION OF RETINA.
  $\boxed{\text{a-wave}}$ -choroidal circulation $\boxed{\text{b-wave}}$ -retinal circulation

CONDITIONS:
- PIGMENTARY RETINOPATHY
- CONGENITAL STATIONARY NIGHT BLINDNESS
- CENTRAL RETINAL ARTERY OCCLUSION ⎫ Negative ERG
- RETINOSCHISIS ⎭ Absent b-wave

NB:
- oscillatory response abnormal in EARLY (pre-proliferate) DIABETIC RETINOPATHY

PERG – Pattern ERG

- Alternating Black and White checks followed by reverse pattern (2–6 Hz)

Amplitude(μV)

- P_{50} • Probably GANGLION CELL origin
- N_{95} • GANGLION CELL ORIGIN
- Secondary phenomenon to P_{50}

USE:
- CENTRAL RETINA - MACULA/GANGLION CELLS
- Further interpretation of VEP (- Glaucoma, Ocular Hypertension)

CONDITIONS:
- MACULOPATHY – Abnormal P_{50}
  – Normal N_{95}/P_{50} ratio
- OPTIC NEUROPATHY
  - Abnormal N_{95}, Normal P_{50}
  - Retrograde ganglion cell degeneration

Conclusion

INVESTIGATION PATHWAY

- Delayed Pattern VEP – Optic Nerve/Macular pathalogy
- PERG Abnormal P50 – Macular pathology
- Abnormal ERG – Peripheral retinal pathology
- Abnormal EOG – RPE pathology

Essay Structure 6 cont.

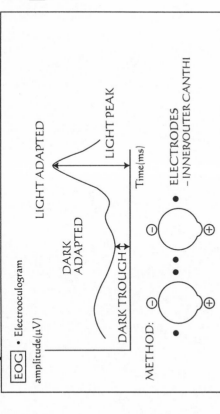

EOG • Electrooculogram

amplitude(μV)

LIGHT ADAPTED

LIGHT PEAK

DARK
ADAPTED

DARK TROUGH↕

Time (ms)

ELECTRODES
– INNER/OUTER CANTHI

METHOD:

- Record Fixed -30° Lateral eye movements at regular intervals during both DARK ADAPTATION and then LIGHT ADAPTATION (approx. 15 min each)
- Principle: Recording corneo-retinal potential
- Minimum signal in dark = DARK TROUGH (DT)
- Maximum signal in light = LIGHT PEAK (LP)
- ARDEN INDEX = $\frac{LP}{DT}$ (≥170% Normal)

USE: RPE - PHOTORECEPTOR INTERACTION
CONDITION: • PIGMENT RETINOPATHY
- METABOLIC/TOXIC CONDITIONS AFFECTING
  RPE. (Choroidal circulation)

Useful- • BESTS DISEASE (VITELLIFORM MACULAR DYSTROPHY)
- Abnormal EOG even in asymptomatic carriers
- REDUCED EOG, NORMAL ERG
- Apical membrane of RPE affected

Essay Structure 7: *Describe the Pathway from the Retina to the Visual Cortex of an Image in the Left Superior Visual Field (Including Retinotopic Organisation)*

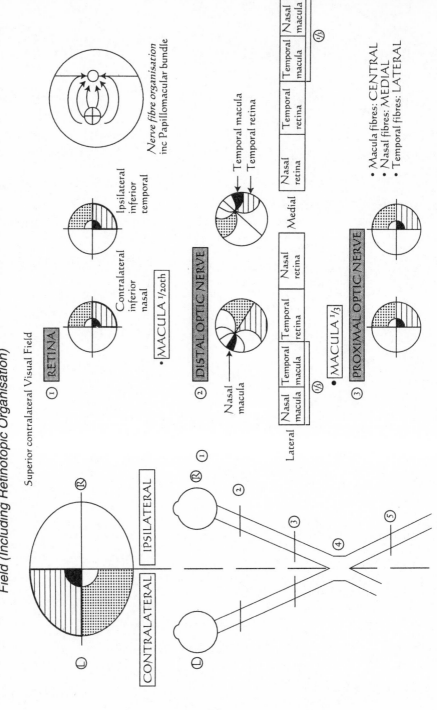

ANTERIOR CHIASM

POSTERIOR CHIASM

④ OPTIC CHIASMA

- Ipsilateral Temporal fibres: UNCROSSED — Inferior retinal: fibres
- Contralateral Nasal fibres: CROSSED — Superior retinal: fibres

⑤ DISTAL OPTIC TRACE

- Contralateral Nasal/Ipsilateral Temporal retina.
- 90° inward twist.
- Superior retinal fibres: MEDIAL.
- Inferior retinal fibres: LATERAL.
- Macular fibres gradually surface.

⑥ LGN

- Contralateral Nasal fibres: LAYERS 1, 4, 6.
- Ipsilateral Temporal fibres: LAYERS 2, 3, 5.
- Macular fibres: DORSAL.
- Superior retinal fibres: VENTROMEDIAL LGN.
- Inferior retinal fibres: DORSOLATERAL LGN.

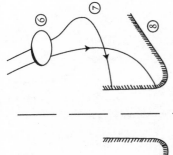
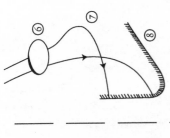

⑦ OPTIC RADIATION

- Superior retinal fibres:

  RADIATION
  - Superior fibres.
  - Run directly posteriorly.
  - To superior lip of Calcarine Sulcus.

- Inferior retinal fibres:
  - Inferior fibres.
  - Swing out Laterally.
  - Inferolateral to Anterior tip of Temporal horn of Lateral Ventricle.
  - Turn inwards to inferior lip of Calcarine Sulcus.

⑧ VISUAL CORTEX

1 cm

- Receives Ipsilateral Temporal/contralateral Nasal retina.
- Superior retinal fibres: SUPERIOR LIP CALCARINE SULCUS.
- Inferior retinal fibres: INFERIOR LIP CALCARINE SULCUS.
- Macular fibres: POSTERIOR 1 cm.

Essay Structure 8: *Give an Account of the Origin, Course, Relations and Functions of the Third Cranial Nerve*

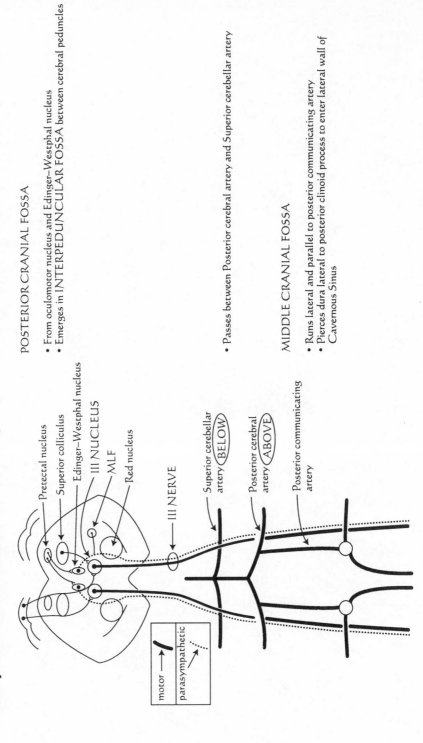

POSTERIOR CRANIAL FOSSA

- From oculomotor nucleus and Edinger–Westphal nucleus
- Emerges in INTERPEDUNCULAR FOSSA between cerebral peduncles

- Passes between Posterior cerebral artery and Superior cerebellar artery

MIDDLE CRANIAL FOSSA

- Runs lateral and parallel to posterior communicating artery
- Pierces dura lateral to posterior clinoid process to enter lateral wall of Cavernous Sinus

Pretectal nucleus
Superior colliculus
Edinger–Westphal nucleus
III NUCLEUS
MLF
Red nucleus

III NERVE

Superior cerebellar artery (BELOW)
Posterior cerebral artery (ABOVE)
Posterior communicating artery

motor →
parasympathetic →

- Initially, high in lateral wall of cavernous sinus
- Then descends medial to IV and V_a
- Receives proprioceptive fibres from V_a (mesencephalic nucleus)
- Receives sympathetic fibres from Internal carotid plexus

- Divides into *Superior* and *Inferior* divisions

- Enters orbit through Superior Orbital fissure within the common tendinous ring

SUPERIOR DIVISION – Runs lateral to optic N
           – Runs below Superior Rectus
           – Pierces Superior Rectus
           – Supplies LEVATOR with • MOTOR and
                              • SYMPATHETIC fibres Internal Carotid plexus

INFERIOR DIVISION – Lies above Inferior Rectus and Inferior Oblique
           – Supplies • PARASYMPATHETIC fibres to ciliary
                     ganglion (inferolateral to Optic Nerve)

FUNCTION • Supplies Superior Rectus/• Levator (inc. SYMPATHETIC fibres)
              • Supplies Medial Rectus
              • Supplies Inferior Rectus/• Inferior Oblique
              • Supplies preganglionic parasympathetic fibres to ciliary ganglion
          →postganglionic parasympathetic supply to sphincter pupillae and ciliary muscle

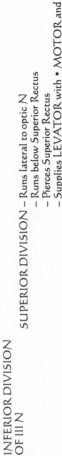

III
IV
V_a
V_b
VI

SUPERIOR DIVISION OF III N
INFERIOR DIVISION OF III N

Lacrimal N
Frontal N
IV
Nasociliary N
VI

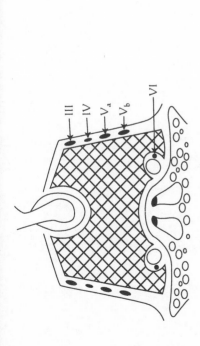

SUPERIOR DIVISION
LEVATOR
SR
Short ciliary nerves
IO
INFERIOR DIVISION
IR
Ciliary ganglion

Essay Structure 9: *Give an Account of the Origin, Course, Relations and Function of the Fourth Cranial Nerve*

- From *Trochlear Nucleus* – dorsal midbrain, just below inferior colliculus

- Decussate
- Emerge posteriorly

- Pass lateral to Superior cerebellar peduncle – around lateral aspect of midbrain

- Runs between posterior cerebral artery and superior cerebellar artery

- Pierces dura near posterior clinoid process

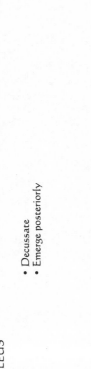

inferior colliculus

IV NUCLEUS

MLF

Tectobulbar
from superior colliculus

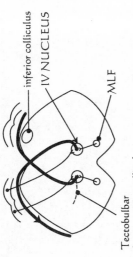

Posterior
view

MIDBRAIN

Superior cerebellar
peduncle

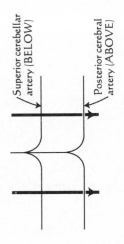

Superior cerebellar
artery (BELOW)

Posterior cerebral
artery (ABOVE)

- Enters lateral wall of Cavernous Sinus
- Crossed medially by descending III nerve

- Enters orbit through superior orbital fissure OUTSIDE and SUPEROLATERAL to common tendinous ring

- Passes medially above Levator muscle
- Terminates in superior surface of superior oblique muscle
- FUNCTION: - Motor fibres to superior oblique muscle

    Intorsion
    Depression
    Lateral rotation

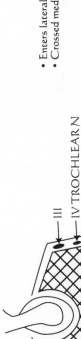

III
IV TROCHLEAR N
V_a
V_b
VI

"Luscious
Fancy } LFT
Tarts
Sit
Naked
In
Anticipation"

Abducent N VI

Lacrimal N
Frontal N
IV TROCHLEAR NERVE
Superior division of III N
Nasociliary N
Inferior division of III N

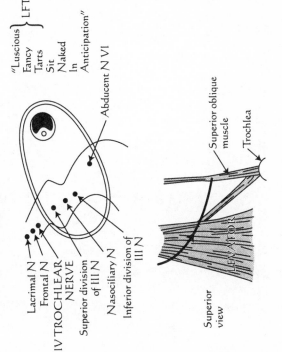

Superior oblique muscle
Trochlea

LEVATOR

Superior view

Essay Structure 10: Give an Account of the Origin, Course, Relations and Functions of the Sixth Cranial Nerve

- Floor of IVth Ventricle
- Beneath facial colliculus
- Emerges from anterior brainstem
- Pontomedullary junction

- Runs
  - Forwards
  - Upwards
  - Laterally in subarachnoid space

- Crosses over tip of petrous temporal bone
  (Anchored by reflection of dura – Petrospheroidal ligament of Gruber
  – resembling a canal = Dorello's Canal)

- Pierces dura inferolateral to dorsum sellae

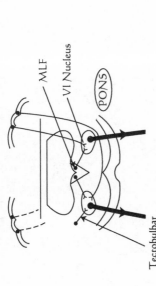

MLF

VI Nucleus

PONS

Tectobulbar
from superior
colliculus

PONS

medulla

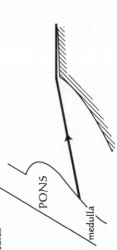

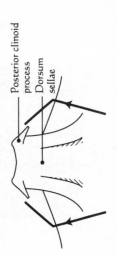

POSTERIOR CRANIAL FOSSA

Posterior clinoid
process
Dorsum
sellae

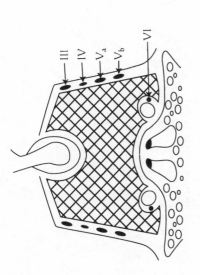

- Runs within cavernous sinus lateral to internal carotid artery

III
IV
V$_a$
V$_b$
VI

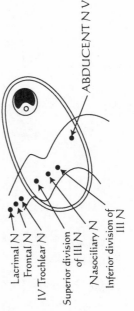

- Passes into orbit through superior orbital fissure,
  – within common tendinous ring – inferomedially
- Passes forward to enter medial surface of lateral rectus muscle

- FUNCTION – motor supply to lateral rectus muscle which rotates the eye laterally

ABDUCENT N VI

Lacrimal N
Frontal N
IV Trochlear N

Superior division
of III N

Nasociliary N

Inferior division of
III N

Essay Structure 11: *Describe the Mechanisms of Visual Adaptation*

INTRO:

LIGHT SENSE
= • Awareness of light and modifications of its intensity

INTENSITY
Due to • light source • object reflectance

BRIGHTNESS
• Measured in unit of luminance (L)
• Candela/m²
• Photometric unit
• Radiance (radiometric) corrected for spectral efficiency of standardized eye

VISUAL ADAPTATION
= • Phenomenon of automatic adjustment of visual sensitivity to changes in illumination

MAIN:

Eye functions in both bright sunlight and starlight, yet sunlight has 10 billion times greater intensity than starlight

IMPORTANCE OF VISUAL ADAPTATION
• Visual perception is based on LOCAL CONTRAST rather than ambient levels of illuminance
  → LATERAL INHIBITION and ON/OFF RETINAL CHANNELS
• Visual system must detect both DARK and LIGHT spots in order to register an image
• Therefore, better to respond to changes in LIGHTER areas
• Ambient dark-to-light can be 10^9-fold intensity change

• Between ROD-DEPENDENT and CONE-DEPENDENT vision

CHANGE IN QUALITY OF VISION

Changes in:
① TEMPORAL ACUITY
② VISUAL ACUITY - spatial resolution
③ SPECTRAL SENSITIVITY → 'PURK(IN)JE SHIFT'

ROD-DEPENDENT VISION
max. sensitivity at blue light
CONE-DEPENDENT VISION
max. sensitive at Red/Green light

• RANGE = 0 – 9 log units (increase in threshold from absolute threshold)

• Sensitivity = $\dfrac{1}{\text{threshold}}$

LIGHT ADAPTATION

To • ↓ sensitivity
 • Extract contrast

PUPIL SIZE

• Takes up to [1 second]
• Reduce light input by
 [1 log unit] = 10 – 30 fold

NB: Unit of [Retinal] illuminance
= TROLAND (T)
= Illuminance (L) × pupil area (P)
 (mm^2)

RETINAL NEURAL ACTIVITY

• Takes [milliseconds]
• Range [3 log units]

• LATERAL INHIBITION
 – Horizontal/Amacrine Cells
• ON/OFF RETINAL CHANNELS
 – Bipolar/Ganglion/LGN/?Cortex

HORIZONTAL CELL FEEDBACK THEORY

• Alter gain control
• [LIGHT] → [CONE] → [HORIZONTAL CELL]
 Hyperpolarize Hyperpolarize

Depolarize [CONES] → [TO ALTER GAIN]
and Delay

• Significant effect with [Large diffuse] light stimulus, causing [BRIEFER AND SMALLER CONE RESPONSE] than for small spot of light

• Horizontal Cell [EMPHASIZES] spatially [DISCRETE/SPOT?] stimuli

PHOTOCHEMICALS

• Takes [Seconds to minutes]
• Range [8 log units]

• Altered steady state concentration of photosensitive pigments

Photochemicals and photosensitive pigments ⇌ Retinaldehyde & opsins ↕ Vitamin A (LIGHT)

• Poorly understood molecular basis:
 ↓[CGMP] → ↓[Ca^{2+}] intracellular
 'internal messenger'

• ↓[PHOTOCHEMICALS] ↑ → ↓ SENSITIVITY

NB: 10% Bleached photopigment cause 100-fold sensitivity loss.

Essay Structure 11 cont.

DARK ADAPTATION

|e.g. Exposure to total darkness after several hours of bright light|

PUPIL SIZE – above

RETINAL NEURAL ACTIVITY – above

PHOTOCHEMICALS

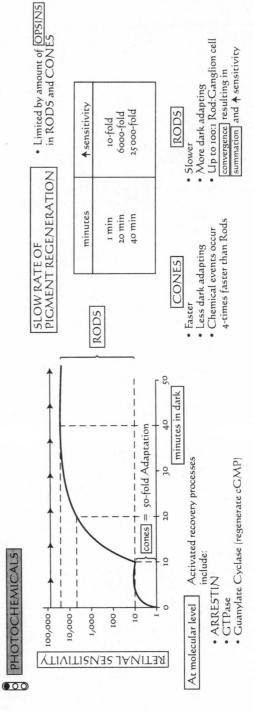

- Limited by amount of **OPSINS** in RODS and CONES

SLOW RATE OF PIGMENT REGENERATION

minutes		sensitivity
1 min		10-fold
20 min		6000-fold
40 min		25 000-fold

CONES
- Faster
- Less dark adapting
- Chemical events occur 4-times faster than Rods

RODS
- Slower
- More dark adapting
- Up to 100:1 Rod:Ganglion cell convergence resulting in summation and ↑ sensitivity

RODS

cones = 50-fold Adaptation

minutes in dark

RETINAL SENSITIVITY

100,000
10,000
1,000
100
10
1

At molecular level — Activated recovery processes include:
- ARRESTIN
- GTPase
- Guanylate Cyclase (regenerate cGMP)

CONCLUSION:
- 3 Main mechanisms
- Mainly at Retinal level
- Speed vs Range
- Important for extraction of local contrast

Essay Structure 12: *Describe the Control of Pupillary Responses and its Modifications by Drugs*

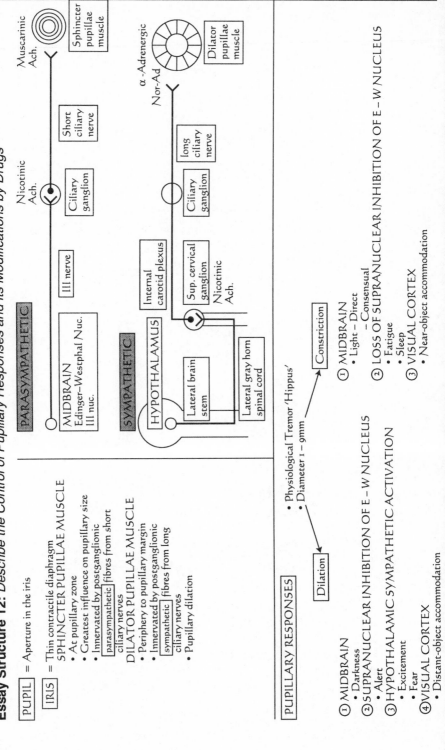
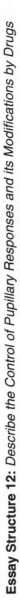

PUPIL = Aperture in the iris

IRIS = Thin contractile diaphragm

SPHINCTER PUPILLAE MUSCLE
- At pupillary zone
- Greatest influence on pupillary size
- Innervated by postganglionic parasympathetic fibres from short ciliary nerves

DILATOR PUPILLAE MUSCLE
- Periphery to pupillary margin
- Innervated by postganglionic sympathetic fibres from long ciliary nerves
- Pupillary dilation

PARASYMPATHETIC

Muscarinic Ach.

Sphincter pupillae muscle

Nicotinic Ach.

Short ciliary nerve

Ciliary ganglion

III nerve

MIDBRAIN
Edinger–Westphal Nuc.
III nuc.

SYMPATHETIC

α-Adrenergic Nor-Ad

Dilator pupillae muscle

long ciliary nerve

Ciliary ganglion

Internal carotid plexus

Sup. cervical ganglion
Nicotinic Ach.

HYPOTHALAMUS

Lateral brain stem

Lateral gray horn spinal cord

PUPILLARY RESPONSES
- Physiological Tremor 'Hippus'
- Diameter 1 – 9mm

Dilation

① MIDBRAIN
- Darkness

② SUPRANUCLEAR INHIBITION OF E – W NUCLEUS
- Alert

③ HYPOTHALAMIC SYMPATHETIC ACTIVATION
- Excitement
- Fear

④ VISUAL CORTEX
- Distant-object accommodation

Constriction

① MIDBRAIN
- Light – Direct
      – Consensual

② LOSS OF SUPRANUCLEAR INHIBITION OF E – W NUCLEUS
- Fatigue
- Sleep

③ VISUAL CORTEX
- Near-object accommodation

MODIFICATION BY DRUGS   • Act at synapses – peripherally
                                                                – centrally

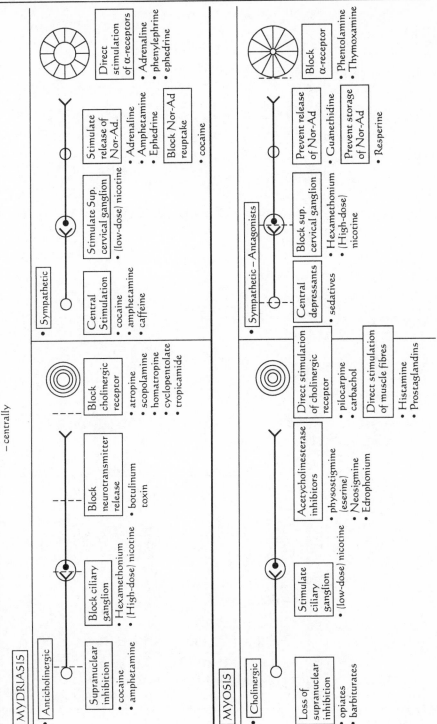

MYDRIASIS

• Anticholinergic

| Supranuclear inhibition |
• cocaine
• amphetamine

| Block ciliary ganglion |
• Hexamethonium
• (High-dose) nicotine

| Block neurotransmitter release |
• botulinum toxin

| Block cholinergic receptor |
• atropine
• scopolamine
• homatropine
• cyclopentolate
• tropicamide

• Sympathetic

| Central Stimulation |
• cocaine
• amphetamine
• caffeine

| Stimulate Sup. cervical ganglion |
• (low-dose) nicotine

| Stimulate release of Nor-Ad. |
• Adrenaline
• Amphetamine
• Ephedrine

| Block Nor-Ad reuptake |
• cocaine

| Direct stimulation of α-receptors |
• Adrenaline
• phenylephrine
• ephedrine

MYOSIS

• Cholinergic

| Loss of supranuclear inhibition |
• opiates
• barbiturates

| Stimulate ciliary ganglion |
• (low-dose) nicotine

| Acetycholinesterase inhibitors |
• physostigmine (eserine)
• Neosigmine
• Edrophonium

| Direct stimulation of cholinergic receptor |
• pilocarpine
• carbachol

| Direct stimulation of muscle fibres |
• Histamine
• Prostaglandins

• Sympathetic – Antagonists

| Central depressants |
• sedatives

| Block sup. cervical ganglion |
• Hexamethonium
• (High-dose) nicotine

| Prevent release of Nor-Ad |
• Guanethidine

| Prevent storage of Nor-Ad |
• Reserpine

| Block α-receptor |
• Phentolamine
• Thymoxamine

ESSAY STRUCTURE 13: *DISCUSS THE ANATOMICAL AND PHYSIOLOGICAL BASIC OF BINOCULAR VISION*

INTRO:

Definition:

| BINOCULAR VISION | = Use of both eyes simultaneously |
| BINOCULAR SINGLE VISION | = Use of both eyes for common single perception (Develops after birth) |

Key Terms: ① Retinal Correspondence ② Horopter ③ Panum's Area ④ Stereopsis ⑤ Diplopia

① RETINAL CORRESPONDENCE

- Both eyes have some valid direction
- Point on nasal retina in one eye corresponds to point on temporal retina in the other eye during binocular vision

  Nasal Retina ⟶ Temporal field (vice versa)

③ STEREOPSIS

- Perception of relative depth
- Relies on binocular disparity
- Object lies in Panum's space

④ PANUM'S SPACE AND AREA

Panum's Area
- Non-corresponding points *on retina* that allow fusion

Panum's Space
- Space around Horopter where slightly non-corresponding points are seen as *single with depth*
- Smallest at fixation point
- Increases in periphery

② HOROPTER

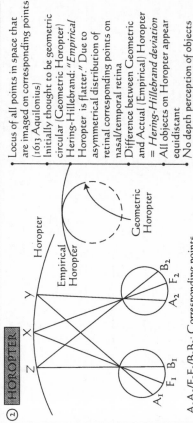

- Locus of all points in space that are imaged on corresponding points (1613 Aquilonius)
- Initially thought to be geometric circular (Geometric Horopter)
- Hering-Hillebrand: *"Empirical Horopter is flatter."* Due to asymmetrical distribution of retinal corresponding points on nasal/temporal retina
- Difference between Geometric and Actual (Empirical) Horopter = *Hering-Hillebrand deviation*
- All objects on Horopter appear equidistant
- No depth perception of objects on Horopter (No disparity)

$A_1A_2/F_1F_2/B_1B_2$: Corresponding points

⑤ DIPLOPIA

Pathological
- Deviation of one eye from fixation point

Physiological
- Objects in front of, or behind Horopter/Panum's space
  Crossed/Heteronymous: Near-object diplopia
  Uncrossed/Homonomous: Far-object diplopia
  Normally SUPPRESSED to allow binocular single vision

MAIN:
• Evidence at level of RETINA LGN VISUAL CORTEX

(Historical) TYPES OF BINOCULAR VISION (Worth 1903)
• Simple Classification

① SIMULTANEOUS PERCEPTION
Perception of two separate images

② FUSION

Sensory
Two images seen and interpreted as one image

Motor
• Maintenance of sensory fusion by Vergence → Horizontal / Vertical / Cyclovergence

③ STEREOSCOPIC FUSION
• Perception of two slightly different images and interpretation as one image with DEPTH

① RETINA
Topographical organization (Retinal Correspondence)
Transferred by parallel channels from:
photoreceptor -- bipolar cell -- ganglion cell -- LGN --Vis. Cortex.
($M \to P$ cells)

② LGN

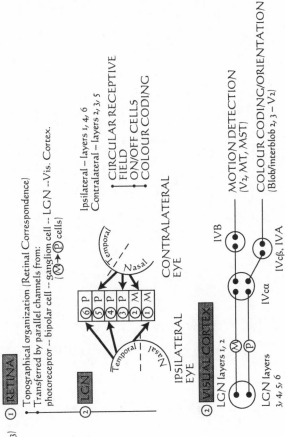

Temporal
Nasal
IPSILATERAL EYE

6 P
5 P
4 P
3 M
2 M
1 M

Temporal
Nasal
CONTRALATERAL EYE

Ipsilateral – layers 1, 4, 6
Contralateral – layers 2, 3, 5

CIRCULAR RECEPTIVE FIELD
ON/OFF CELLS
COLOUR CODING

② VISUAL CORTEX

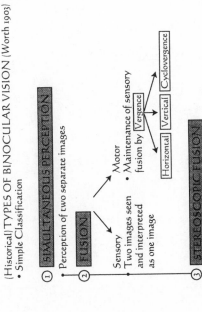

LGN layers 1, 2 — IVB
LGN layers 3, 4, 5, 6 — IVcα, IVcβ, IVA

MOTION DETECTION (V2, MT, MST)
COLOUR CODING/ORIENTATION (Blob/interblob 2, 3 – V2)

• Layer IV – incoming signals are MONOCULAR (from each eye)
• Layer II, III, V, VI – converge to BINOCULAR CELLS
• BINOCULAR CELLS • Sensitive to disparity (non-corresponding points)
• Driven by each eye

(In research stage):
Parvocellular: Tuned Near, Tuned Far, Tuned zero, Tuned inhibitory
Magnocellular: Near and Far neurones
• Majority of Striate cells are binocular
• Able to detect disparity
• Able to maintain alignment (magnocellular MOTION DETECTION) – VERGENCE

ESSAY STRUCTURE 13 cont.

THEORIES OF BINOCULAR VISION AND FUSION

PHYSIOLOGICAL

- Due to BLENDING of two images
  Based on anatomy/physiology of virtual pathway:
  Eyes have overlapping visual fields
  Retinal correspondence (including size, colour and brightness)

- Partial decussation at optic chiasm, therefore, each visual cortex codes for contralateral visual field
  Binocular cells at visual cortex
  EXPLAINS: STEREOPSIS
- Fusion of retinal image disparity

ALTERNATING SUPPRESSION

- Due to alternating suppression of each image
  (Alternating suppression of
    • Corresponding points
    • Use of each eye)

- Never simultaneous binocular perception
- e.g. Asher (1953) "RETINAL RIVALRY"

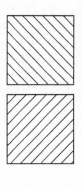

Gobin (1971) "MOSAIC VIEWING"
Point sampling of information in field

EXPLAINS: SINGLE IMAGE PERCEPTION

Essay Structure 14: *Discuss the Factors Governing Penetration of Drugs into the Eye*

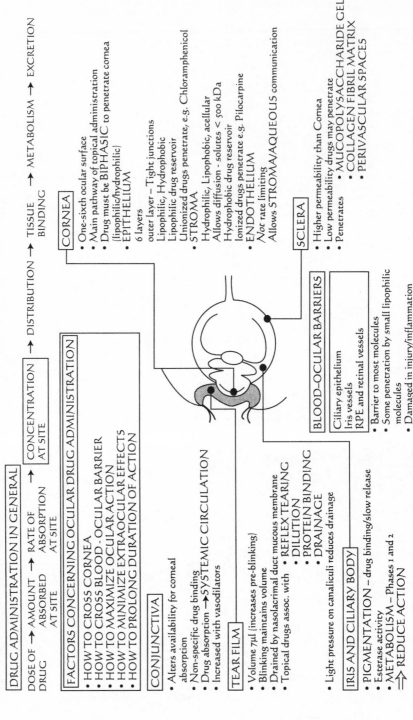

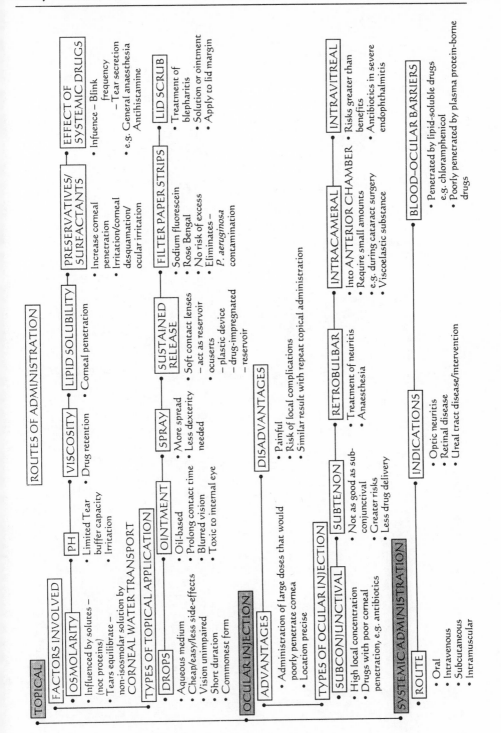

ROUTES OF ADMINISTRATION

TOPICAL

FACTORS INVOLVED

OSMOLARITY
• Influenced by solutes –
  (not proteins)
• Tears equilibrate –
  non-isosmolar solution by
  CORNEAL WATER TRANSPORT

PH
• Limited Tear
  buffer capacity
• Irritation

VISCOSITY
• Drug retention

LIPID SOLUBILITY
• Corneal penetration

PRESERVATIVES/
SURFACTANTS
• Increase corneal
  penetration
• Irritation/corneal
  desquamation/
  ocular irritation

EFFECT OF
SYSTEMIC DRUGS
• Influence – Blink
              frequency
            – Tear secretion
• e.g. General anaesthesia
        Antihistamine

TYPES OF TOPICAL APPLICATION

DROPS
• Aqueous medium
• Cheap/easy/less side-effects
• Vision unimpaired
• Short duration
• Commonest form

OINTMENT
• Oil-based
• Prolong contact time
• Blurred vision
• Toxic to internal eye

SPRAY
• More spread
• Less dexterity
  needed

SUSTAINED
RELEASE
• Soft contact lenses
  – act as reservoir
• ocuserts
  – plastic device
  – drug-impregnated
    – reservoir

FILTER PAPER STRIPS
• Sodium fluorescein
• Rose Bengal
• No risk of excess
• Eliminates –
  P. aeruginosa
  contamination

LID SCRUB
• Treatment of
  blepharitis
• Solution or ointment
• Apply to lid margin

OCULAR INJECTION

ADVANTAGES
• Administration of large doses that would
  poorly penetrate cornea
• Location precise

DISADVANTAGES
• Painful
• Risk of local complications
• Similar result with repeat topical administration

TYPES OF OCULAR INJECTION

SUBCONJUNCTIVAL
• High local concentration
• Drugs with poor corneal
  penetration, e.g. antibiotics

SUBTENON
• Not as good as sub-
  conjunctival
• Greater risks
• Less drug delivery

RETROBULBAR
• Treatment of neuritis
• Anaesthesia

INTRACAMERAL
• Into ANTERIOR CHAMBER
• Require small amounts
• e.g. during cataract surgery
• Viscoelastic substance

INTRAVITREAL
• Risks greater than
  benefits
• Antibiotics in severe
  endophthalmitis

SYSTEMIC ADMINISTRATION

ROUTE
• Oral
• Intravenous
• Subcutaneous
• Intramuscular

INDICATIONS
• Optic neuritis
• Retinal disease
• Ureal tract disease/intervention

BLOOD–OCULAR BARRIERS
• Penetrated by lipid-soluble drugs
  e.g. chloramphenicol
• Poorly penetrated by plasma protein-borne
  drugs

Essay Structure 15: *Outline the Blood Supply to the Visual Pathway*

Intro:

• Retina ——→ Optic Nerve ——● Optic Chiasma ——● Optic Tract ——● LGN ——● Optic radiation ——● Visual Cortex

• Internal Carotid Artery ←——→ Circle of Willis ←——→ Basilar Artery

Pathway:

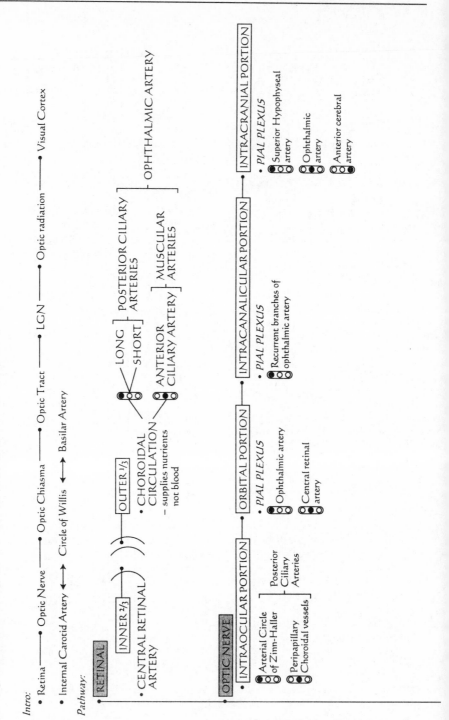

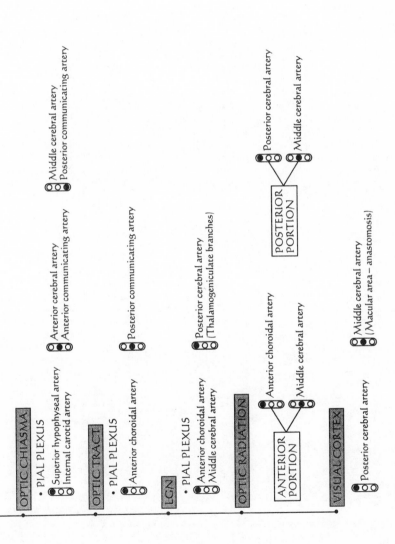

OPTIC CHIASMA
• PIAL PLEXUS
  • Superior hypophyseal artery
  • Internal carotid artery
    • Arterior cerebral artery
    • Anterior communicating artery
      • Middle cerebral artery
      • Posterior communicating artery

OPTIC TRACT
• PIAL PLEXUS
  • Anterior choroidal artery
    • Posterior communicating artery

LGN
• PIAL PLEXUS
  • Anterior choroidal artery
  • Middle cerebral artery
    • Posterior cerebral artery
    • (Thalamogeniculate branches)

OPTIC RADIATION
ANTERIOR PORTION
  • Anterior choroidal artery
  • Middle cerebral artery
POSTERIOR PORTION
  • Posterior cerebral artery
  • Middle cerebral artery

VISUAL CORTEX
  • Posterior cerebral artery
    • Middle cerebral artery
    • (Macular area – anastomosis)

CONCLUSION:
• INTERNAL CAROTID ARTERY – Main supply to Retina – optic radiation
• BASILLAR ARTERY – Main supply to Optic radiation – Visual Cortex

Essay Structure 16: *Describe the Causes and Effects of Ulcers*

DEFINITION: Disruption in the continuity of an EPITHELIAL surface resulting from the sloughing of necrotic inflammatory material

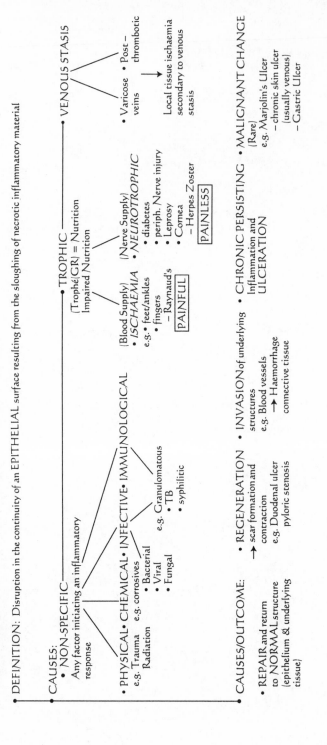

CAUSES:
- NON-SPECIFIC
  Any factor initiating an inflammatory response

- PHYSICAL • CHEMICAL • INFECTIVE • IMMUNOLOGICAL
  e.g. Trauma   e.g. corrosives   • Bacterial   e.g. Granulomatous
       Radiation   • Viral   • TB
                                    • Fungal   • syphilitic

                                    TROPHIC
                                    (Trophé/GR) = Nutrition
                                    Impaired Nutrition

  (Blood Supply)   (Nerve Supply)
  • ISCHAEMIA   • NEUROTROPHIC
  e.g. feet/ankles   • diabetes
    • fingers   • periph. Nerve injury
    – Raynaud's   • Leprosy
  PAINFUL   • Cornea
                                – Herpes Zoster
                              PAINLESS

                                    VENOUS STASIS
                              • Varicose   • Post –
                                veins   thrombotic

                                    Local tissue ischaemia
                                    secondary to venous
                                    stasis

CAUSES/OUTCOME:

- REPAIR and return
  to NORMAL structure
  (epithelium & underlying
  tissue)

- REGENERATION
  → scar formation and
    contraction
    e.g. Duodenal ulcer
    pyloric stenosis

- INVASION of underlying
  structures
  e.g. Blood vessels
    → Haemorrhage
    connective tissue

- CHRONIC PERSISTING
  Inflammation and
  ULCERATION

- MALIGNANT CHANGE
  (Rare)
  e.g. Marjolin's Ulcer
    – chronic skin ulcer
    (usually venous)
    – Gastric Ulcer

EXAMPLES

- PEPTIC ULCERATION
"Ulcer in an acid-secreting area"

- Acid
- Pepsin

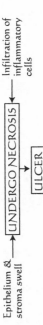

Protective mechanisms
- mucus
- pH gradient
- Tight junctions
- Rapid Regeneration
- $PGE_2 - \uparrow$ mucus $\downarrow$ acid
- HCO_3^-

Aetiology:
- Helicobacter pylori – 95% D.U., 75% G.U.

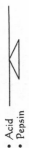
- acute gastritis
- inflammatory response
- $\downarrow$ protection

- NSAIDs – PGE_2, G.U. only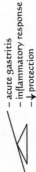
- Autoimmune Gastritis (pernicious anaemia)
- Rare = Z–E, Crohn's, Stress –? Cephalic stimulation of acid production

Complications:
- Scarring → Pyloric stenosis 'BLOCK'
- Haemorrhage 'BLEED'
- Perforation → peritonitis 'BURST'
- Adherence + erosion – pancreas, liver
- Malignant change

- CORNEAL ULCERS

Epithelium & stroma swell → UNDERGO NECROSIS ← Infiltration of inflammatory cells
↓
ULCER

type:
- CENTRAL assoc. with:
  - pneumococcal/Strep/Staph – primary infection
  - Hypopyon – cloudy sterile exudate in anterior chamber
  - Anterior/posterior synechiae

- MARGINAL *(periphery)*

  SIMPLE
  - Associated with blepharoconjunctivitis
  - Usually due to staphylococcal toxin

  RING
  - Peripheral ulcers, coalesce circumferentially
  - Associated with PAN, LE, Wegeners', R.A.
  - Due to Scleral connective tissue disease/vasculitis

- MOOREN'S
  - Elderly
  - Bilateral, shallow ulcer
  - Unknown aetiology

- DENDRITIC (Branch-like)
  - e.g. Herpes simplex
  - Associated with stromal keratitis

SEQUELAE:
- OPACITY – scarring
- ECTATIC CICATRIX/KERATECTASIA – scar bulges out
- DESCEMETOCOELE – Ulceration leaves Descemet's membrane only, bulges out due to I.O.P.
- PERFORATION – Rupture of cornea, possible prolapse of iris and lens
- ANTERIOR STAPHYLOMA – Prolapsed iris and tissue epitheliazes bulges out due to I.O.P.

Essay Structure 17: *Discuss the Genetic Mechanisms Involved in Neoplasia*

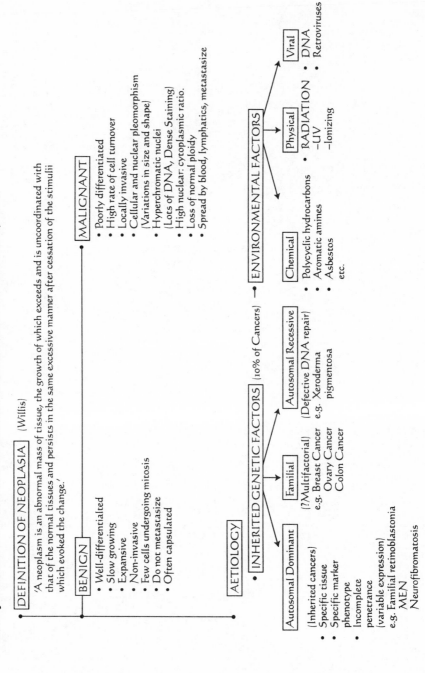

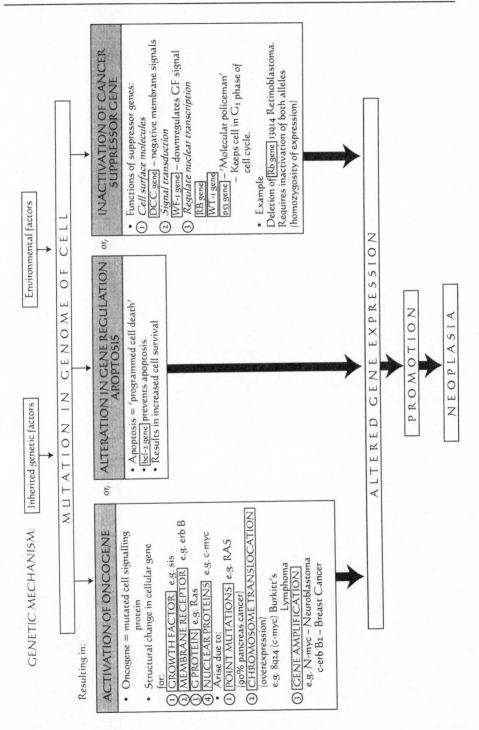

GENETIC MECHANISM:

Inherited genetic factors

Environmental factors

MUTATION IN GENOME OF CELL

Resulting in:

ACTIVATION OF ONCOGENE
- Oncogene = mutated cell signalling protein
- Structural change in cellular gene for:
  - ① GROWTH FACTOR e.g. sis
  - ② MEMBRANE RECEPTOR e.g. erb B
  - ③ G PROTEIN e.g. Ras
  - ④ NUCLEAR PROTEINS e.g. c-myc
- Arise due to:
  - ① POINT MUTATIONS e.g. RAS (90% pancreas cancer)
  - ② CHROMOSOME TRANSLOCATION (overexpression)
    e.g. 8q24 (c-myc) Burkitt's Lymphoma
  - ③ GENE AMPLIFICATION
    e.g. N-myc – Neuroblastoma
    c-erb B2 – Breast Cancer

or,

ALTERATION IN GENE REGULATION APOPTOSIS
- Apoptosis = 'programmed cell death'
- bcl-2 gene prevents apoptosis
- Results in increased cell survival

or,

INACTIVATION OF CANCER SUPPRESSOR GENE
- Functions of suppressor genes:
  - ① Cell surface molecules
    DCC gene – negative membrane signals
  - ② Signal transduction
    WT-1 gene – downregulates GF signal
  - ③ Regulate nuclear transcription
    RB gene
    WT-1 gene
    p53 gene – 'Molecular policeman'
    – Keeps cell in G_1 phase of cell cycle.
- Example
  Deletion of Rb gene 13q14 Retinoblastoma.
  Requires inactivation of both alleles (homozygosity of expression)

ALTERED GENE EXPRESSION

PROMOTION

NEOPLASIA

Essay Structure 18: *Discuss the Possible Local and Systemic Effects of Neoplasia*

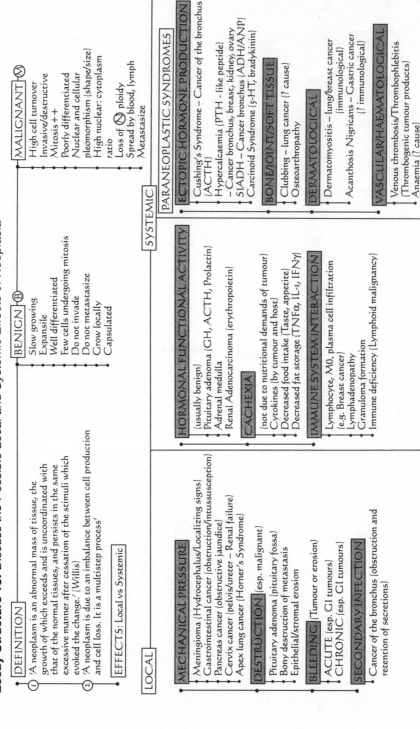

DEFINITION

① 'A neoplasm is an abnormal mass of tissue, the growth of which exceeds and is uncoordinated with that of the normal tissues, and persists in the same excessive manner after cessation of the stimuli which evoked the change.' (Willis)

② 'A neoplasm is due to an imbalance between cell production and cell loss. It is a multistep process'

EFFECTS: Local vs Systemic

BENIGN Ⓑ
- Slow growing
- Expansile
- Well differentiated
- Few cells undergoing mitosis
- Do not invade
- Do not metastasize
- Grow locally
- Capsulated

MALIGNANT Ⓜ
- High cell turnover
- Invasive/destructive
- Mitosis + +
- Poorly differentiated
- Nuclear and cellular pleomorphism (shape/size)
- High nuclear: cytoplasm ratio
- Loss of Ⓝ ploidy
- Spread by blood, lymph
- Metastasize

LOCAL

MECHANICAL PRESSURE
- Meningioma (Hydrocephalus/Localizing signs)
- Gastrointestinal cancer (obstruction/intussusception)
- Pancreas cancer (obstructive jaundice)
- Cervix cancer (pelvis/ureter – Renal failure)
- Apex lung cancer (Horner's Syndrome)

DESTRUCTION (esp. malignant)
- Pituitary adenoma (pituitary fossa)
- Bony destruction of metastasis
- Epithelial/stromal erosion

BLEEDING (Tumour or erosion)
- ACUTE (esp. GI tumours)
- CHRONIC (esp. GI tumours)

SECONDARY INFECTION
- Cancer of the bronchus (obstruction and retention of secretions)

SYSTEMIC

HORMONAL FUNCTIONAL ACTIVITY
- (usually benign)
- Pituitary adenoma (GH, ACTH, Prolactin)
- Adrenal medulla
- Renal Adenocarcinoma (erythropoietin)

CACHEXIA
- (not due to nutritional demands of tumour)
- Cytokines (by tumour and host)
- Decreased food intake (Taste, appetite)
- Decreased fat storage (TNFα, IL-1, IFNγ)

IMMUNE SYSTEM INTERACTION
- Lymphocyte, M0, plasma cell infiltration (e.g. Breast cancer)
- Lymphadenopathy
- Granuloma formation
- Immune deficiency (Lymphoid malignancy)

PARANEOPLASTIC SYNDROMES

ECTOPIC HORMONE PRODUCTION
- Cushing's Syndrome – Cancer of the bronchus (ACTH)
- Hypercalcaemia (PTH - like peptide) – Cancer bronchus, breast, kidney, ovary
- SIADH – Cancer bronchus (ADH/ANP)
- Carcinoid Syndrome (5-HT, bradykinin)

BONE/JOINT/SOFT TISSUE
- Clubbing – lung cancer (? cause)
- Osteoarthropathy

DERMATOLOGICAL
- Dermatomyositis – lung/breast cancer (immunological)
- Acanthosis Nigricans – Gastric cancer (? immunological)

VASCULAR/HAEMATOLOGICAL
- Venous thrombosis/Thrombophlebitis (Thrombogenic tumour products)
- Anaemia (? cause)

Essay Structure 19: Discuss with Appropriate Examples the Causes and Effects of Ischaemia

DEFINITION: State of inadequate arterial perfusion to organ tissue relative to metabolic needs

INCIDENCE: Common!

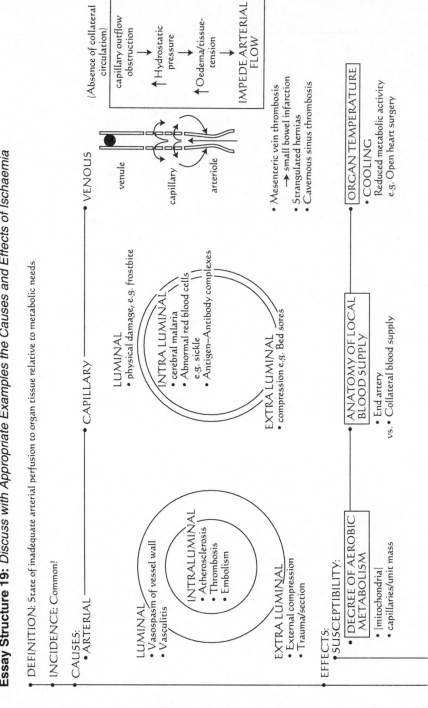

CAUSES:
- ARTERIAL ———————————— CAPILLARY ——————————— VENOUS

LUMINAL
- Vasospasm of vessel wall
- Vasculitis

INTRALUMINAL
- Atherosclerosis
- Thrombosis
- Embolism

EXTRALUMINAL
- External compression
- Trauma/section

LUMINAL
- physical damage, e.g. frostbite

INTRALUMINAL
- cerebral malaria
- Abnormal red blood cells
  e.g. sickle
- Antigen–Antibody complexes

EXTRALUMINAL
- compression e.g. Bed sores

venule

capillary

arteriole

(Absence of collateral circulation)
capillary outflow obstruction
↓
↑ Hydrostatic pressure
↓
↑ Oedema/tissue-tension
↓
IMPEDE ARTERIAL FLOW

- Mesenteric vein thrombosis → small bowel infarction
- Strangulated hernias
- Cavernous sinus thrombosis

EFFECTS:
SUSCEPTIBILITY:

- DEGREE OF AEROBIC METABOLISM
  - ↓mitochondrial
  - capillaries/unit mass

- ANATOMY OF LOCAL BLOOD SUPPLY
  - End artery
  vs. Collateral blood supply

- ORGAN TEMPERATURE
  - COOLING
    Reduced metabolic activity
    e.g. Open heart surgery

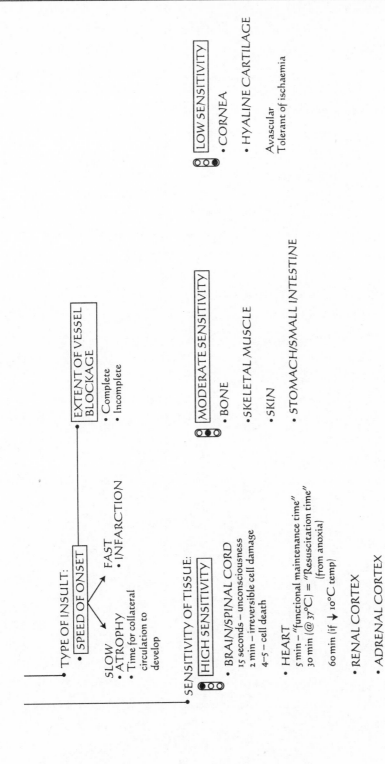

TYPE OF INSULT:

• SPEED OF ONSET

SLOW
• ATROPHY
• Time for collateral
  circulation to
  develop

FAST
• INFARCTION

EXTENT OF VESSEL
BLOCKAGE
• Complete
• Incomplete

SENSITIVITY OF TISSUE:

HIGH SENSITIVITY

• BRAIN/SPINAL CORD
  15 seconds – unconsciousness
  2 min – irreversible cell damage
  4–5 – cell death

• HEART
  5 min – "functional maintenance time"
  30 min (@ 37°C) = "Resuscitation time"
  (from anoxia)
  60 min (if ↓ 10°C temp)

• RENAL CORTEX

• ADRENAL CORTEX

MODERATE SENSITIVITY

• BONE

• SKELETAL MUSCLE

• SKIN

• STOMACH/SMALL INTESTINE

LOW SENSITIVITY

• CORNEA

• HYALINE CARTILAGE

Avascular
Tolerant of ischaemia

Essay Structure 20: *Describe the Causes and Effects of Occlusive Disease Occurring in Muscular Arteries and Arterioles Including Gross and Microscopic Pathology*

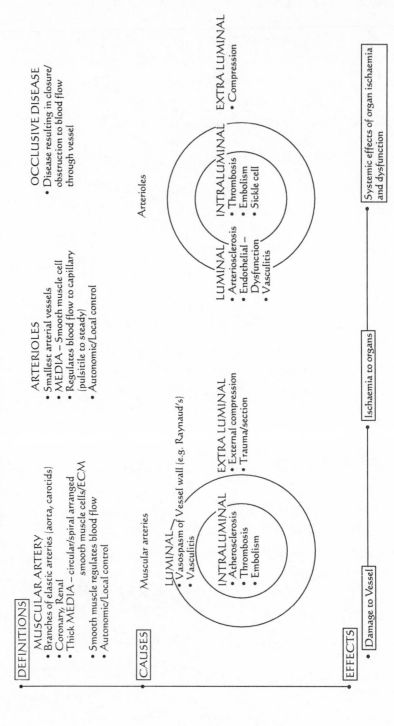

DEFINITIONS

MUSCULAR ARTERY
- Branches of elastic arteries (aorta, carotids)
- Coronary, Renal
- Thick MEDIA – circular/spiral arranged smooth muscle cells/ECM
- Smooth muscle regulates blood flow
- Autonomic/Local control

ARTERIOLES
- Smallest arterial vessels
- MEDIA – Smooth muscle cell
- Regulates blood flow to capillary (pulsitile to steady)
- Autonomic/Local control

OCCLUSIVE DISEASE
- Disease resulting in closure/obstruction to blood flow through vessel

CAUSES

Muscular arteries

LUMINAL
- Vasospasm of Vessel wall (e.g. Raynaud's)
- Vasculitis

INTRALUMINAL
- Atherosclerosis
- Thrombosis
- Embolism

EXTRA LUMINAL
- External compression
- Trauma/section

Arterioles

LUMINAL
- Arteriosclerosis
- Endothelial – Dysfunction
- Vasculitis

INTRALUMINAL
- Thrombosis
- Embolism
- Sickle cell

EXTRA LUMINAL
- Compression

EFFECTS

- Damage to Vessel → Ischaemia to organs → Systemic effects of organ ischaemia and dysfunction

DETAILS:

ATHEROSCLEROSIS

- Proliferative intimal disease
- Involving medium/large muscular/elastic arteries
- Associated with Hypercholesterolaemia
  Hypertension
  Smoking
  Diabetes

GROSS
- Raised focal intimal atheroma (fibrofatty plaque)
- Associated with FATTY STREAKS (yellow; at bifurcations)

MICROSCOPIC (core)
- Lipid
- Collagen
- Smooth muscle cells
- Macrophages
- +/- T cell immune reaction

EFFECTS
- Occlusive in SMALL ARTERIES (ischaemia)
- Destructive in LARGE ARTERIES (Aneurysm, rupture, risk thrombosis)

Examples:
- Chronic ischaemic heart disease (coronary)
- Gangrene of leg (popliteal)
- CVA (cerebral)
- Acute occlusive thrombosis (Ulceration of atherosclerotic plaque, and exposure of subendothelial connective tissue)

THROMBOSIS

- Solid mass/plug from components of blood in a living blood vessel (or heart)

VIRCHOW'S TRIAD:
- Changes in Intimal vessel surface
  e.g. Atherosclerosis
       Acute vasculitis
       Trauma
- Changes in pattern of blood flow
- Changes in constituents of blood

- Occurs in:
  Heart, arteries, capillaries and veins

- Occlusive in arteries
  coronary, cerebral, femoral

GROSS/MICROSCOPIC
- Firmly attached to wall
- Fibrin/platelet mesh of clot

EFFECTS
- Acute/chronic occlusion
  (myocardial infarction, chronic ischaemic heart disease)
- CVA (cerebral arteries)
- Embolism

EMBOLISM

- Abnormal mass, solid, gaseous, liquid, carried in blood stream and impacts in vessel lumen too small to allow it to pass
- 99%: Thromboembolic

- 1% include:
  Atheromatous plaque
  Bone
  Fat
  Air
  Nitrogen etc.

Effect
- Occlusion/ischaemia/+/- infarction

Variable Factors:
- Tissue affected/state of tissue
- Size of embolus
- Blood supply (end artery/collaterals)
- Temperature etc.

Sites of impaction:
- 75% Lower limbs
- 10% Brain
- 10% Mesenteric, Renal, Splenic
- 5% Upper limbs

Essay Structure 20 cont.

ARTERIOLES:

ATHERIOSCLEROSIS
- Proliferation/Hyaline thickening
- Seen especially in kidney arterioles

ASSOCIATED WITH:
Hypertension – Benign (Thickening/Hyalinization of wall)
– Malignant
  Haemorrhages
  Fibrinoid necrosis
  Intimal hyperplasia
  Thrombosed capillaries

Diabetes

EFFECTS
Narrow lumen
Ischaemia/infarct distally

VASCULITIS
- Large vessel disease (Giant cell arteritis, Takayasu's)
- Medium vessel disease (Giant cell, PAN, Kawasaki)
- Small vessel disease (Giant cell, Wegener's, Buerger's)
- Inflammation/+/– Necrosis of blood vessel

CAUSE:
INFECTIVE
IMMUNOLOGICAL
- Immune complex deposition
- ANCA-C (cytoplasmic) – Wegener's
- ANCA-P (perinuclear) – PAN, Glomerular disease
- Antibody-mediated (Goodpasture's Anti-BM)
- Cell-mediated (Allograft rejection)

UNKNOWN (Giant cell arteritis)

GROSS/MICROSCOPIC
Intimal fibrosis, thickening, hyperplasia
Leukocyte infiltration/+/– granuloma/+/– Necrosis (focal/diffuse)

PAN – Bifurcations, localized, aneurysms
– Fibrinoid necrosis
– Healed areas: Transmural scarring

Thromboarteritis obliterans (Buerger's disease)
Acute/chronic inflammation
small arteries
segmental occlusive thrombosis
(? Tobacco hypersensitivity)

Raynaud's Phenomenon
NB (Raynaud's disease = idiopathic)
Secondary to arterial narrowing
SLE, Scleroderma, atherosclerosis, Buerger's

EFFECTS
Endothelial dysfunction/Activation
Thrombosis (distal ischaemia/infarction)

ENDOTHELIAL DYSFUNCTION
Response to abnormal stimulus
Modifies normal function
Expression of new properties
SPECTRUM OF DISEASE:

ENDOTHELIAL ACTIVATION
Hours/days, Protein synthesis
cytokine production
Loss of heparin-like surface-molecules
Tissue factor expression

- Spasm
- Thrombosis
- OCCLUSION

ENDOTHELIAL STIMULATION
Rapid, reversible
e.g. Histamine → CONTRACTION

EFFECTS:
Intimal hyperplasia
Fibrin deposition
Decreased release EDRF
Increased abnormal vasoconstriction

Essay Structure 21: *Describe the Absorption of Ultra Violet, Visible and Infrared Light by the Eye. Discuss Their Harmful Effects*

INTRO:

LIGHT
• Visual system sensitive to electromagnetic portion of spectrum

ENERGY
• Light energy $\propto \dfrac{1}{\text{wavelength}}$
• Photon of BLUE light has TWICE the energy as a photon of RED light

SUN
• Radiant source
• 1% energy sustains life on earth

OZONE
• 2.4–4.6 mm THICK LAYER
• Absorbs UV peak @ 290 nm
• Very little UV below 300 nm reaches Earth

TYPES OF RADIATION	WAVELENGTH (nm) $10^{12} - 10^{6}$	PHOTON ENERGY (eV) 0.001	EFFECT OF ABSORPTION
Long wave, Medium wave, Shortwave, Microwave			Heating (Rotation and Vibration)
SUN { INFRARED	$760 - 10^{5}$	≤ 1	Excitation heating and molecular dissociation
VISIBLE	$400 - 760$	2	
ULTRAVIOLET }	$200 - 400$	$3 - 6$	
Xray-radiation, Gamma-radiation	$1 - 10^{-2}$	12	Ionization (Bonds broken)

ULTRAVIOLET LIGHT
• Most damaging light radiation

UV-A
• 320–400 nm
• PHOTOSENSITIZING EFFECT

UV-B
• 290–320 nm
• Absorbed by nucleic acid etc.
• ALTERS FUNCTIONAL MOLECULES
  – nucleic acids/proteins

UV-C
• 200–290 nm
• Does not reach Earth (OZONE)
• DAMAGES DNA/NUCLEIC ACIDS

ABSORPTION IN EYE

CORNEA
• UV-B
• Infrared >1400 nm

ANTERIOR CHAMBER
• Infrared – Melanin (Iris and Trab. Meshwork)

LENS
• UV-A

RETINA – PIGMENTS
• LIGHT – Photoreceptor pigments
• Infrared – Melanin (RPE)
  – Xanthophyll (macula)

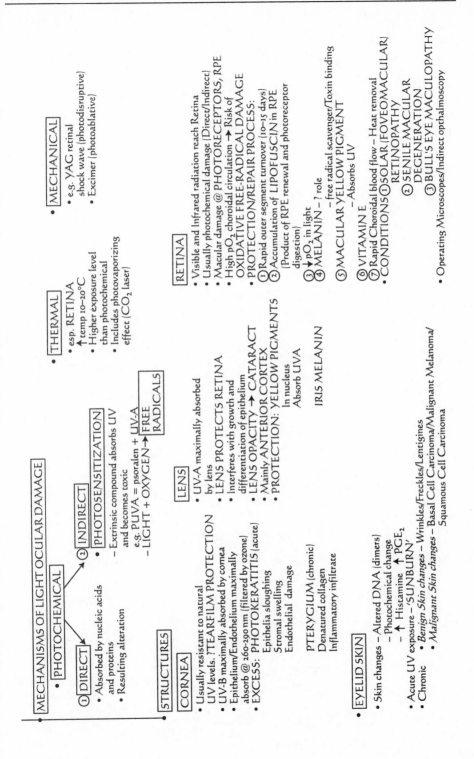

MECHANISMS OF LIGHT OCULAR DAMAGE

• PHOTOCHEMICAL

① DIRECT
- Absorbed by nucleic acids and proteins
- Resulting alteration

② INDIRECT

PHOTOSENSITIZATION
- Extrinsic compound absorbs UV and becomes toxic
  - e.g. PUVA = psoralen + UV-A
  - LIGHT + OXYGEN → **FREE RADICALS**

• THERMAL
- esp. RETINA
  - ↑ temp 10–20°C
- Higher exposure level than photochemical
- Includes photovaporizing effect (CO_2 laser)

• MECHANICAL
- e.g. YAG retinal shock wave (photodisruptive)
- Excimer (photoablative)

STRUCTURES

CORNEA
- Usually resistant to natural UV levels. ?TEARFILM PROTECTION
- UV-B maximally absorbed by cornea
- Epithelium/Endothelium maximally absorb @ 260–290 nm (filtered by ozone)
- EXCESS: PHOTOKERATITIS (acute)
  - Epithelia sloughing
  - Stromal swelling
  - Endothelial damage

  PTERYGIUM (chronic)
  - Denatured collagen
  - Inflammatory infiltrate

LENS
- UV-A maximally absorbed by lens
- LENS PROTECTS RETINA
- Interferes with growth and differentiation of epithelium
- LENS OPACITY → CATARACT
  - Mainly ANTERIOR CORTEX
- PROTECTION: YELLOW PIGMENTS
  In nucleus
  Absorb UVA

  IRIS MELANIN

RETINA
- Visible and Infrared radiation reach Retina
- Usually photochemical damage (Direct/Indirect)
- Macular damage @ PHOTORECEPTORS, RPE
- High pO_2 choroidal circulation → Risk of OXIDATIVE FREE-RADICAL DAMAGE
- PROTECTION/REPAIR PROCESS:
  ① Rapid outer segment turnover (10–15 days)
  ② Accumulation of LIPOFUSCIN in RPE (Product of RPE renewal and photoreceptor digestion)
  ③ → pO_2 in light
  ④ MELANIN – ? role
    – free radical scavenger/Toxin binding
  ⑤ MACULAR YELLOW PIGMENT
    – Absorbs UV
  ⑥ VITAMIN E
  ⑦ Rapid Choroidal blood flow – Heat removal
- CONDITIONS ① SOLAR (FOVEOMACULAR) RETINOPATHY
  ② SENILE MACULAR DEGENERATION
  ③ BULL'S EYE MACULOPATHY
- Operating Microscopes/Indirect opthalmoscopy

EYELID SKIN
- Skin changes – Altered DNA (dimers)
  – Photochemical change
  – ↑ Histamine ↑ PGE_2
- Acute UV exposure – 'SUNBURN'
- Chronic • Benign Skin changes – Wrinkles/Freckles/Lentigines
  • Malignant Skin changes – Basal Cell Carcinoma/Malignant Melanoma/Squamous Cell Carcinoma

BIBLIOGRAPHY

Adler, FH (1992) *Adler's physiology of the eye*, 9th edn, ed. WM Hart, Mosby Yearbook.

Arden, GM, ed. (1972) *The visual system – neurophysiology, biophysics and their clinical application*, Plenum Press.

Cotran, RS, Kumar, V and Robbins, SL (1994) *Robbins' pathologic basis of disease*, 5th edn, Saunders.

Davison, H, *Physiology of the eye*, Churchill Livingstone.

Duane, TD and Jaeger, EA, *Duane's foundations of ophthalmology*, Lippincott–Raven.

Ganong (1993) *Medical physiology*, 16th edn, Appleton & Lang.

Gardner, DL and Tweedle, DEF (1996) *Pathology for surgeons in training*, Edward Arnold.

Gray, H (1995) *Gray's anatomy*, 38th edn, Churchill Livingstone.

Guyton (1991) *Textbook of medical physiology*, 8th edn, Saunders.

Kanski, J (1994) *Clinical ophthalmology*, 3rd edn, Butterworth–Heinemann.

Kumar, PJ (1994) *Clinical medicine*, Baillière Tindall.

Last, RJ (1994) *Last's anatomy*, 9th edn, Churchill Livingstone.

Lehninger, AL (1982) *Principles of biochemistry*, Worth.

Lowenstein, O and Loewenfeld, IE (1969) *The pupil*, Academic Press.

Maisel, H, ed. (1985) *The ocular lens: structure, function and pathology*, Marcel Dekker.

Miller, SJH, *Parson's diseases of the eye*, 17th edn.

Regan, D (1989) *Human brain electrophysiology – evoked potentials and evoked magnetic fields in science and medicine*, Elsevier.

Roitt, IM (1994) *Essential immunology*, 8th edn, Blackwell Science.

Saude, T (1993) *Ocular anatomy and physiology*, Blackwell Science.

Seal, DV, 'Acanthamoeba Keratitis', *British Medical Journal*, 308, 1116–17.

Sleigh, JD and Timbury, MC (1994), *Medical bacteriology*, 4th edn, Churchill Livingstone.

Snell, RS and Lemp, MA (1989) *Clinical anatomy of the eye*, Blackwell.

Spillman, L and Werner, JS, eds (1990) *Visual perception*, Academic Press.

Whikehart, DR (1994) *Biochemistry of the eye*, Butterworth–Heinemann.

Wolff, E (1968) *Eugene Wolff's anatomy of the eye and orbit including the central connections, development and comparative anatomy of the visual apparatus*, 6th edn, ed. RJ Last, HK Lewis.

Woolf, N (1986) *Cell, tissue and disease*, 2nd edn, Baillière Tindall.

INDEX OF QUESTION TOPICS